ZOONOSES and the ORIGINS and ECOLOGY of HUMAN DISEASE

ZOONOSES
and the ORIGINS and ECOLOGY
of HUMAN DISEASE

by

Richard N. T-W-Fiennes

1978

ACADEMIC PRESS

London   New York   San Francisco

A Subsidiary of Harcourt Brace Jovanovich, Publishers

ACADEMIC PRESS INC. (LONDON) LTD.
24/28 Oval Road,
London NW1

United States Edition published by
ACADEMIC PRESS INC.
111 Fifth Avenue
New York, New York 10003

Library of Congress Catalog Card Number: 77 93212
ISBN: 0 12 256050 7

PRINTED IN GREAT BRITAIN BY THE LAVENHAM PRESS LIMITED
LAVENHAM SUFFOLK

To John and Maura

Preface

The purpose of this book is not to give a catalogue of animal diseases, from which man can suffer; rather, the human disease pattern is reviewed in relation to ecology—the relationships of man with his environment and with the animals with which he associates. In the penultimate chapter, the part played in human disease by marine biology is briefly discussed, since it is likely to become increasingly important and has not hitherto been evaluated.

It is evident that the human disease pattern has changed fundamentally since populations became increasingly concentrated in towns and cities. A number of entirely new diseases have appeared, not shared with any kind of animal, which require minimal population densities for survival. Many such diseases must have arisen from pathogens of animal origins, which have become adapted to man as the sole host. In this sense, they are "remote zoonoses". There is also evidence that this trend in disease evolution is by no means past, and that "new" or new sub-types of existing diseases are still becoming adapted to the human host.

The emergence of new diseases could well result in pandemic episodes which could kill a great many people in many parts of the world before control could be effected. World conditions today resemble those which in the past have preceded the appearance of global pandemics and the dangers should be realised.

This book, then, does not supersede existing works on zoonoses, which are of high merit and cover the field comprehensively. It does seek to expand the areas of thought on the subject, in ways which appear, to the author, to be of fundamental importance. This importance is emphasised by study of the part played by suddenly-appearing new diseases on human history, the course of which has been changed as a result at various times for better or for worse.

References have, in so far as possible, been limited to general articles and books on the subject in question. Current thought on the influenza problem has been so recently developed, that I have needed personal guidance and assistance. This has been readily accorded, and I wish to acknowledge my debt to Dr. G. C. Schild of the Medical

Research Council Influenza Unit, and to Professor W. I. B. Beveridge and Dr. Abdusalam of the World Health Organization.

NOVEMBER, 1978   RICHARD FIENNES
111 Gloucester Court,
Kew Gardens,
Richmond,
Surrey

Introduction

Introduction

On May 14th 1796, Edward Jenner inoculated a boy named James Phipps with fluid from a vesicle on the finger of a dairy maid, Sarah Nelmes. Sarah had contracted cowpox from the udder of a cow that she had been milking. Neither Sarah nor the cow were at all sick, except for the inconvenience of local lesions on the skin of finger and udder. Jenner was testing the age-old belief in the West Country that persons, who had suffered from cowpox, did not contract smallpox. On July 1st of the same year, he administered to James vesicle material from a smallpox case. James did not contract smallpox, nor did 22 other persons on whom Jenner subsequently tried his technique.

Today, there would no doubt be an outcry from humanitarian societies, broadcast through the mass media, at Jenner's inhumanity in exposing the boy to the danger of contracting a deforming and often fatal disease. There was no such outcry, but members of the medical profession were frankly disbelieving and obstructed the introduction of vaccination. It was, at the time, common practice to infect exposed persons deliberately with small inoculations of smallpox material in the hope that the resulting disease would be milder than if naturally acquired; it did not, therefore, seem so outrageous for Jenner to infect the boy as might appear today.

These events occurred fifty years before Koch and Pasteur, and before the infectious nature of disease had been demonstrated. The Great Plague of 1665 had occurred only 131 years before and was believed to be wafted by the southern wind and due to poisonous vapours. It was fifty years later that Chadwick removed the handle from the Fleet pump, convinced that contamination of the water supply was the cause of cholera. Life expectation was short; early death and all manner of tragedy were accepted with resignation and ascribed to the will of God.

The well known story of Jenner and the cowpox is of interest for a number of reasons. Long before there was any understanding of the infectious causes of disease he did, on an empirical basis, find a means of protecting people from one of the most serious. It is interesting, because he proceeded on the basis of an "old wives' tale", though why the old wives had not long since ensured that everybody suffered from cowpox is difficult to discern except by acceptance of the divine will.

It is also interesting in our context, because the disease from which Sarah Nelmes was suffering was a "zoonosis"; it was a disease of cattle, which could be transmitted to human beings, in this case in a very mild form as in the cattle. It appears to have been recognised that people did contract disease from animals, though this recognition was probably confined to obvious cases such as cowpox, in which the connection could not very well be overlooked. Disease cycles involving intermediate hosts were not only unrecognised but seemed so absurd as to be laughable. That acute observer, the explorer Richard Burton, mentioned in his "First Footsteps in East Africa" the belief amongst Somali tribesmen that malaria was somehow connected with mosquitos, a belief — so he thought — typical of primitive people whose society was riddled with superstition. Even so, the Philistines in the days of King Hezekiah of Judah seem to have recognised the connection of plague with rodents, since when pestilence fell on them they appeased the god of Israel by offerings of golden mice. Furthermore, the connection of dirt and lice with outbreaks of typhus was certainly understood in a vague sort of way.

Etymology

When preparing my book "Zoonoses of Primates", I was prompted to undertake some research into the origin of the word "zoonoses"; it seemed to me that the word was in frequent use, but nobody seemed to understand its precise meaning. In this, I was assisted by a German lady, the late Miss E. von Bernuth, and the results appear more fully in my book. The use of the term had appeared in German and French medical lexicons by the middle of the nineteenth century. For example, Probstmayer (1863) in his "Dictionary of Veterinary Medicine" defined zoonoses as: — "Zoonoses are firstly original animal diseases; secondarily, diseases of man which can be transmitted to him by means of a contagion from animals." Evidently, the term had been in use for some length of time before finding its way into the dictionaries. British scientists have attributed the word to the great German pathologist, Virchow (1821-1902), in the belief that he had coined it. This, however, is not the case; Miss Bernuth, in spite of a careful search of his writings, could discover no instance in which he used the term other than in a strictly orthodox way as defined above. In its strict sense the term means merely an animal disease in man, or indeed simply an animal disease.

The concept then was originally without subtlety and seems to have fallen into disuse until after the Second World War. During the past twenty years, it has come into its own again particularly in tropical medicine, because of the realisation that so many diseases are passed, in one way or another, between animal and man and because they are so important. Zoonoses have thus become a new and fascinating branch of medical science in their own right. They could hardly have become so, until a knowledge had been acquired of transmissible pathogens and of the intricacies of disease cycles. Inevitably, the term zoonosis has acquired a wider meaning and indeed has become a new science.

Like all new sciences, that of zoonoses has tended to acquire a terminology of its own, most of it unnecessary and some of it etymologically unsound. Thus, if a zoonosis is an animal disease transmissible to man, what is a human disease transmissible to an animal? This difficulty was solved by introducing the term "anthro ponosis". If these two terms are accepted, another term is necessary for diseases from which both animals and man can suffer and which can be passed in either direction from one to the other. This problem gave rise to the term "amphixenosis", which is meaningless in terms of its Greek derivations. There are also terms such as "anthropozoonosis" and "zooanthroponosis". Even further into the realms of fantasy are terms such as protozoonosis and helminthozoonosis, meant to mean protozoan and helminth diseases transmissible from animals to man, but which literally mean diseases of protozoa and helminths from which man can also suffer.

These terms are all best discarded with the possible exception of anthroponosis, though there is little necessity even for this. We are concerned with the dangers of animal disease to man; the dangers of human diseases for animals, with the possible exception of tuberculosis in monkey colonies, are secondary. In any case, man is a ZOŎN (ζωον) as an animal, so that zoonoses can be used correctly for the two way passage of diseases.

Throughout this work, I use the terms pandemic, epidemic and endemic, whether referring to disease in man and animals. Substitution of the terms panzootic, epizootic and enzootic is both unnecessary and confusing. Reference to Liddell and Scott's Greek Lexicon will show that the greek word "démŏs" (δημοο) can refer to a crowd of either human beings or of animals, although in its derived meaning it usually refers to the former. Primatologists using the English language have difficulty in the use of the word primate, which includes man. Whereas in German the word "affen" and in French "singe" mean both apes and monkeys, there is no word in English to cover both groups, and phrases such as "non-human primates" are commonly used. The late Dr. Hamish Innes suggested that the difficulty could be overcome by using "simian primates" or "simians" for short to cover both apes and monkeys. Purists may object to using the adjective as a noun, but we do the same with "humans"; convenience of expression must prevail. I, therefore, accept Dr. Innes' proposed usage.

Scope and Argument

Since its inception, then, the term zoonosis has been greatly widened, especially by its application to vector-borne diseases. This again present problems as to what may justifiably be regarded as a zoonosis. For example is Yellow Fever a zoonosis? It is a disease which can affect man as well as monkeys, though endemic only in the latter; yet mosquitos are the reservoirs of the virus, and strictly speaking it is not a primate zoonosis but a mosquito zoonosis. Unless we allow some flexibility to the term zoonosis, we find ourselves in difficulty.

These difficulties become greater when, as in this book, one attempts to place zoonoses against a background of disease ecology; in this context, the term zoonosis must be stretched beyond limits which some readers may regard as permissible. There are three main aspects of the subject to be tackled. The first is to study those diseases which are group specific to man, but must have had their origins as zoonoses in the remote past; they are "remote zoonoses", though they are not zoonoses today. Secondly, we study new diseases which may be establishing themselves in man today as a result of his changed ecological circumstances. Thirdly, an account will be given of those diseases derived from animal sources, which create special problems in the modern world. To cover this brief, as I feel it should be covered, I find myself examining the problem of diseases caused by or derived from marine creatures, which do not normally feature in works on zoonoses. If an oyster concentrates the pathogens of typhoid or infectious hepatitis and transmits the disease to a human patient, is this a zoonosis? The dividing line is blurred. When fish are dying as a result of a "red tide" and persons who eat them become sick, they have acquired a disease of fish, a fish zoonosis. If they become sick from eating fish, which have concentrated a heavy metal such as mercury, is this a zoonosis? The Greek word "nŏsŏs" means merely illness or pathology; it does not stipulate that the cause must be a living organism.

I am then using the word zoonosis to cover those aspects of human medical ecology, which depend on man-animal relationships. These relationships are very variable and they have varied greatly throughout history. They differ between Stone Age hunting communities and settled rural and urban communities. They also differ with trades and professions; people who handle animals or animal products are at greater risk than those who do not. The life cycles of parasites are an equally important factor; the connection between a disease of monkeys in the forest and one of human village dwellers, Kyasanur Forest Disease, was not readily apparent until the role of a three host tick was understood; the larvae live on the monkeys in the trees and the nymphs carry infection to cattle and so to the village dwellers. The connection was even more difficult to discover with Yellow Fever in Africa, since the monkeys there show no symptoms when infected. The life cycles of animals which form the disease reservoir must also be taken into account. Some animals migrate seasonally; some hibernate or aestivate; with others there are population explosions every few years when animals overflow their natural boundaries as with lemmings; their natural commensals in stressed conditions cause active symptoms of diseases, such as tularaemia, which prove serious when transmitted to man from his dogs which gorge on the lemmings. Rodents, such as field mice and voles, tend to leave the fields after the harvest and enter human settlements, often introducing infection or contaminating foodstuffs with their faeces.

References

I have then in this work tried to introduce a new angle to the study of zoonoses, which appears to me to be of importance and also of great interest; the material offered is accordingly selective. There are a number of excellent works on zoonoses, which I have used freely to ascertain my facts. Outstanding as a work of reference is van der Hoeden's (1964) "Zoonoses". Another valuable work is Bisseru's (1967) "Diseases of Man acquired from his Pets", which is much more comprehensive than the title might imply. Soulsby's "Parasitic Zoonoses" is invaluable in the field it covers. I have also made reference throughout to a number of works, which I have myself either written or edited, because the material is most readily available in them. The most important of these are: — "Zoonoses of Primates" (Fiennes, 1967) and "Pathology of Simian Primates" (Fiennes, ed. 1972).

The works quoted are fully referenced. I am, however, including a supplementary reference list covering the major publications on Influenza and Transmissible Cancer, although reference to them is not specifically made in the text. Newer concepts of the origins of influenza pandemics are so recent that the literature is unlikely to be widely known, and Beveridge (1977) has not included references in his

"Influenza — the Last Great Plague". The milestones and advances in transmissible cancer research seem to be so little known in Britain, that inclusion of a bibliography may be helpful. Furthermore, I have deliberately covered this subject in the most truncated way possible, because of expressed scepticism about the suggestion made that any form of cancer could prove to have its origins as a zoonosis.

Contents

PART I

The Evolution of Human Diseases
from Animal Counterparts

CHAPTER 1

Man-Animal Relationships

The Human Environment

Man has existed as *Homo* for at least two million years, of which the past 700 000 have comprised the Pleistocene Epoch occupied by the great Ice Age. During the Ice Age, there were four periods of glaciation separated by three interglacial periods, during which the climate became much warmer in northern regions, even sub-tropical. The sequence of glacial and interglacial is shown by Fig. 1 and the extent of the polar ice cap by Fig. 2 (see also Table 1).

The ancestors of modern man were basically ill adapted to life in arctic tundra and could only survive because of their hunting skills, which provided them not only with food but with animal furs for warm clothing; the use of fire also was necessary both for warmth and for cooking foods unsuited to a light tooth apparatus. In the tundra, however, man found an unoccupied ecological niche with abundant resources and no other major predator except wolves, and with a challenge which his high intelligence enabled him to exploit. Most predators hunt by stealth and cannot exploit open habitats, such as the Ice Age offered. Conversely, the special hunting skills developed by both wolves and man were less suited to the forests, which became developed during the warm interglacials and when the Pleistocene Epoch ended some 12 000 years ago. Fossil evidence, as from the great boulder clays of Norfolk, England, show clearly that during the warm intervals of the Ice Age, numbers of both wolves and man decreased greatly and the wolves became much smaller, Fiennes (1976).

The ecological steps and the time sequence, by which forests again encroached on the tundra at the end of the Pleistocene, are described by Cornwall (1959), from whom Table 2 is taken. Man was again forced into retreat, but reacted in a fashion novel in ecological history by attempting to adapt a new and hostile environment to his needs. The consequences both to man and the environment have been

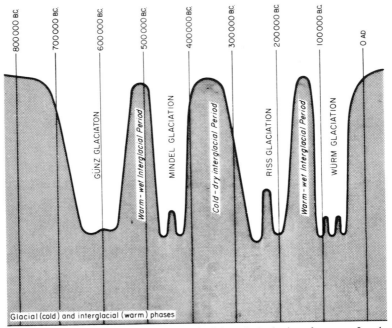

Fig. 1. Sequence of glacial and interglacial periods during the great Ice Age.

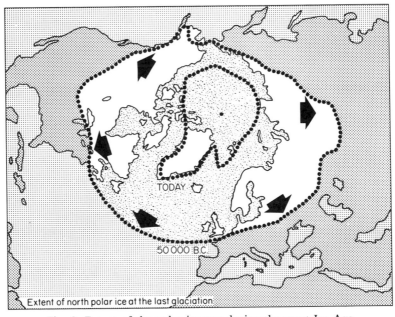

Fig. 2. Extent of the polar ice cap during the great Ice Age.

TABLE 1

Palaeolithic chronology in west and central Europe (After Cornwall, 1959)

Glacial stages	Human artifacts — Cores	Human artifacts — Flakes	Human artifacts — Blades	Years before present
Last Glaciation (Würm) III			Magdalenian Solutrean	25 000
Last Glaciation (Würm) II	Mousterian	Final Levalloisian		72 000
	— Mousterian	Levalloisian V	Aurignacian / Gravettian	
Last Glaciation (Würm) I	Tayacian			115 000
Last Interglacial (Riss-Würm)	Final Acheulian / *Upper Acheulian*			
Penultimate Glaciation (Riss) II	Middle Acheulian	Middle Levalloisian		187 000
Penultimate Glaciation (Riss) I		Early Levalloisian		230 000
Penultimate Interglacial (Mindel-Riss)	Middle Acheulian / Lower Acheulian	*Proto-Levalloisian*		
Antepenultimate Glaciation (Mindel) II		Clactonian II		435 000
Antepenultimate Glaciation (Mindel) 1	Abbevillian (formerly known as Chellean)	Clactonian I		476 000
Antepenultimate Interglacial (Günz-Mindel)	*Cromerian Norwician Ipswician*	Flakes, rostro-carinates, hand-axes		550 000
Early Glaciation (Günz) II	*Abbevillian* (Morocco)			590 000
Early Glaciation (Günz) I		*Sub-Crag Flakes* (E. Anglia)		1 000 000
Villafranchian				

P L E I S T O C E N E

(Uncertainties are printed in italics)

TABLE 2

Late glacial and post-glacial chronology in Scandinavia (After Cornwall, 1959)

Glacial stages — Sweden	Glacial stages — Denmark	Chronology (approx.)	Baltic stages	Climate	Forest history zones	Archaeology
Post-glacial	Post-Glacial		Litorina sea	Sub-Atlantic (cold, wet)	IX Beech	Early Iron Age
		400 B.C.				
			Maxima 4	Sub-Boreal (warm, dry)	VIII Mixed oak forest	Bronze Age / Neolithic
		2500 B.C.	3			
			2	Atlantic (warm, moist, oceanic)	VII Mixed oak forest	Mesolithic
		5000 B.C.	1			
			Ancylus lake	Boreal (warm summers, cold winters; dry, continental)	V, VI Pine and hazel	
		6800 B.C.				
			Yoldia sea	Pre-Boreal (transitional)	IV Birch, pine, willow	
Bipartition of the icesheet Finiglacial retreat Central Swedish moraines	Late Glacial	7900 B.C.				
			Baltic ice-dammed lake	Upper Dryas (sub-Artic)	III Tundra vegetation	
Gotiglacial retreat				Alleröd Stage (warm oscillation)	II Birch and pine	
		9000 B.C.				
South Swedish moraines				Lower Dryas (sub-Artic)	I Tundra vegetation	Upper Palaeolithic

profound, involving amongst other things a complete metamorphosis of human disease patterns and their significance. These changes open a new and somewhat frightening chapter in host-parasite relationships, in which both wild and domestic animals are involved. To understand them, it is first necessary to form some assessment of how diseases affected man at different stages of his emergence into a technological world. This is not an easy task and will involve a degree of guesswork; in some ways it will be easier to indicate, as in Chapter 2, those modern diseases from which man could not formerly have suffered because: —

1. They can only survive at high population densities.
2. Being specific to man, there are no animal reservoirs.

Disease Patterns in Palaeolithic Times

In material terms, the gulf separating modern man from his Palaeolithic ancestors is immense. In terms of geological or evolutionary time, it is insignificant; we are separated by some 400 generations of 30 years and only some 140 life spans of 70 years. Where open hunting grounds persist, Palaeolithic peoples still survive in the Bushmen of the Kalahari in South Africa and in the Australian Aborigines. In so short a time, evolution could not have materially altered the human gene pool and research on fossil material shows that our Cro-Magnon ancestors were inferior to their modern descendants neither in physical development nor in brain size. By some act of evolutionary prescience, the physical and mental capacities to develop an age of technology had been acquired in advance of the need. Only life styles are different.

Knowledge of these life styles comes from archaeological studies of the sites where people lived, and from the study of surviving Palaeolithic peoples. In the first place, they were nomadic, following and hunting the wild animals which provided their food and clothing. In the second place, in spite of being nomadic they possessed some fixed abodes such as caves or rudely constructed dwellings made from mammoth bones or other unlikely materials. Thirdly, they lived and hunted in small communities, consisting of a group of families; they were probably loosely monogamous, but practised "exogamy" or marriage outside the circle of near relatives. Exogamy was assured by the "totem" system, which forbade marriage between two persons of the same totem clan; the system survives in a somewhat debased form to the present in Africa and elsewhere. The people were religious, believing in life after death and propitiating animal gods to assist them in their hunting. In furtherance of the principles of exogamy and for religious veneration, it would appear likely that neighbouring tribes would assemble at certain times of the year such as the winter and summer solstices and the equinoxes.

If these assumptions are correct, then three factors emerge which are relevant in deducing their medical problems: — (i) for most of the year they lived a nomadic life and were part of the tundra ecosystem; infectious diseases would have been of secondary importance to the tribal economy; (ii) for part of the year, they lived in closely confined winter quarters, when there would have been opportunities for diseases to spread but only within the limits of a small band or tribe; (iii) for fixed and limited times, they may have assembled in crowds giving better chances for disease dispersion. This life style is strikingly similar to that of man's fellow tundra predators, the wolves, which live in small family groups in insanitary dens during the summer and follow the wildlife migrations in larger packs during the winter. Disease patterns would conform to those of such a wild predator; commensal resident pathogens would be omnipresent but of little significance, except when conditions became unfavourable or population numbers became excessive. Life expectancy patterns too would have conformed to those of other wild creatures. Two survival curves, the one for animals that were hunted and the other for animals that were not hunted, are given, for comparison with human survival curves for 1798 and 1915 (Figs 3 and 4). The figures show how disease adopted the role of predator in human society, when traditional ways of life were abandoned. Under natural conditions, deaths are high from birth to puberty and again during the approaches to old age. During the intermediate years the numbers of deaths are diminished, except in the hunted community. Palaeolithic man had no natural predators, but lived dangerously because of his hunting activities so that his survival curve may have fallen between the two. Various attempts have been made to estimate longevities of Palaeolithic man relying on the evidence of fossil material. One such, from Deevey (1971), is reproduced in Fig. 5. These figures show a very poor survival rate, but for various reasons such estimates are quite unreliable.

All wild animals carry, or at some time become infected with, potential pathogens, which in early or late life or in stressful conditions may either prove fatal or render a weakened animal an easy prey for predators. Man's later history, furthermore, suggests that he may not have permitted weakly children to survive; he is unlikely to have been averse to cannibalism; and may at times have felt the necessity to sacrifice some members of the community to his gods. In these ways, he may well have taken a hand in adjusting his own population numbers, in effect becoming his own predator.

It is tantalising and frustrating that we cannot glean more accurate information about the ways of life of our ancestors so close in time to ourselves. In a general way, these deductions cannot be too far removed from actuality, and we may attempt to survey the pathogens, which would be present and from time to time important, for comparison with conditions at later dates. These pathogens fall into three main groups: —

1. Usually harmless commensals.

2. Pathogens acquired in youth from other members of the community, which cause illness of limited duration until eliminated or silent.

3. Pathogens acquired from other animals by direct or indirect contact or through intermediate hosts.

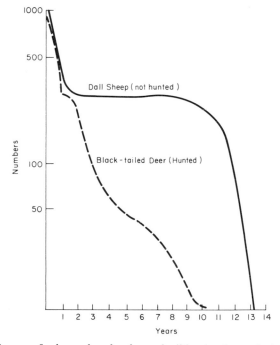

Fig. 3. Survival curves for hunted and unhunted wild animal populations (black-tailed deer and dall sheep). (Compare with chart for survival of human populations in North Germany, in which the curve for 1798 resembles that for the hunted wild population, whereas that for 1915, when hygienic standards of living had been achieved, resembles that for the unhunted wild population.) After Bourlière (1959).

Information about such pathogens can be acquired: — (i) by the study of stone age communities still in existence, such as that by van Amelsfoort (1964); (ii) by the study of fossil skeletal material, *vide* Wells (1964); (iii) by inference from the study of comparable wild living communities; (iv) by study of animal reservoirs of human diseases. A number of the latter will be considered later in this book under such headings as: arboviruses, trypanosomiases, helminthiases.

The most reliable estimate of endemic infections is likely to be that of helminths and other commensals or pathogens of the bowel, since they will have come in unbroken succession from remote times. Such amongst the nematodes, are *Ascaris lumbricoides*, of which a physiological, but morphologically indistinguishable, variant exists in pigs; *Trichuris* and *Enterobius*; *Necator* and *Ancylostoma* amongst the hookworms; and *Strongyloides*. Human *Ancylostoma* is a serious pathogen, if present in large numbers, and closely resembles the *Ancylostoma* of dogs. *Strongyloides* is also pathogenic if present in large numbers; it is rare in temperate climates and closely resembles one of the species found in apes and monkeys. Commensal Protozoa are *Entamoeba coli*, *Iodamoeba*, *Endolimax* and *Isospora*; amongst the pathogens, one would expect *Entamoeba histolytica*, which also infects pigs, *Giardia lamblia*, which infects some herbivores, and *Schistosoma spp.*, which can infect monkeys and of which similar species are present in herbivores, including cattle.

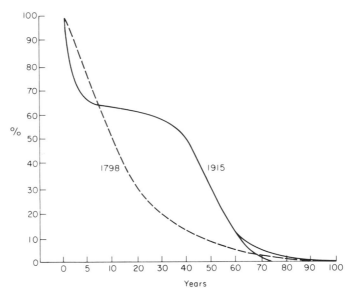

Fig. 4. Survival curves for populations in North Germany. 1. 1798; 2. 1915. (The curve for the 1798 population resembles that for hunted wild animals (Black-tailed Deer); that for 1915 for wild animals that are not hunted (Dall Sheep). The comparison suggests that infectious diseases have adopted the role of predator in the 1798 population. The 1915 human curve, compared with that for the Dall Sheep, shows a prolonged ageing period, which can be attributed to the so-called diseases of senescence, cardiovascular disease and cancer, the onset of which becomes apparent at age 40-50. (After Vischer, 1947).

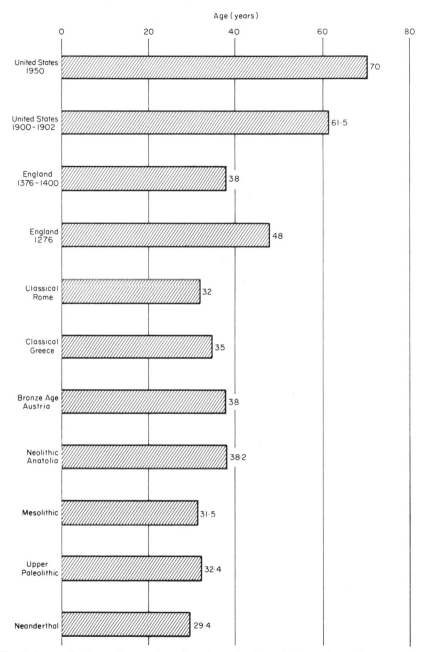

Fig. 5. Longevity in ancient and modern times is charted. From time of Neanderthal man to fourteenth century A.D., life span appears to have hovered around 35 years. An exception is thirteenth-century England. Increase in longevity partly responsible for current population increase has come in modern era. In the U.S. longevity increased about ten years in the last half-century. (From Deevey, 1971).

The common tapeworms of man are *Taenia solium* and *T. saginata*; *T. solium* is acquired by eating the larval form, *Cysticercus cellulosae*, in the flesh of a pig; *T. saginata* is acquired by the consumption of *C. bovis* in beef, but it may also be present in other herbivores. This relationship is clearly derived from the time when man was a hunter, a prey-predator one. The unique nature of the cysticercus larvae suggests a long period of adaptation and evolution and may have originated during Pliocene times before man emerged as *Homo sapiens*. According to Dr. Arthur Bourne (pers. comm.) there may have been a close ecological relationship between man and pigs in the Pliocene, and *C. bovis* could be acquired from reindeer, moose, musk ox or even mammoth. These two cestodes are not normally found in primates other than man. The common cestodes of apes and monkeys are *Bertiella spp.* of the Order Anoplocephalidae acquired by the ingestion of the intermediate hosts, oribatid mites. Persons, who have been in contact with apes or monkeys, sometimes acquire infection but they are not amongst man's normal resident parasites. Human beings, especially children, sometimes become infected with one of the dog tapeworms, *Dipylidium caninum*, which is transmitted by dog fleas.

Association with wolves must also from time to time have resulted in infection from hydatid cysts, which could have proved fatal. Man is not the normal secondary host of this parasite, since wolves rarely, if ever, attack and eat human beings; however, prey meat could easily become contaminated with wolf faeces containing eggs of the adult worm, *Echinococcus granulosus*. One may be sure also that Ice Age peoples would have suffered extensively from trichinosis caused by the nematode *Trichinella spiralis*, acquired today from eating pork. This worm is today widespread in arctic regions, such as Alaska, particularly in bears and Arctic foxes. In tropical countries, man is likely as today to have been host to blood worms of the Order Filaroidea transmitted by arthropod vectors, mosquitos and tabanid biting flies, such as *Chrysops*. The malarias are so host specific that cross-infection with other animals is improbable. However, man was almost certainly universally infected with *Plasmodium ovale*, wherever there was a suitable vector; *P. ovale* is virtually non-pathogenic.

Wild animal reservoirs would also have existed for such diseases as brucellosis, leptospirosis, relapsing fever, salmonelloses, tularaemia, the rickettsioses and plague; the hosts would have been reindeer, other ungulates, rodents, birds, and in tropical regions monkeys. Amongst the viruses, it is well known that in northern regions wolves, especially in times of stress, become infected with rabies, when they will viciously attack human beings. In warmer areas, man would be subject to sporadic infection with arboviruses carried by primates, and everywhere else possibly by bats and other animals.

In company with other creatures living in the wild, man in Palaeolithic times was exposed to many disease hazards, a number of which arose from his association with other animals. It is rare indeed to find no traces of parasitic or other infections macroscopically or microscopically in wild creatures; this I know well from my own researches. Like other animals, man will have lived his life in balance with his pathogens, which only have serious effects at times of ecological imbalance.

Disease Patterns in Mesolithic Times

The recession of the ice at the end of the Pleistocene brought the end of a long period of stability in human history. The speed at which the climate changed is shown in Table 2 above after Cornwall (1959). For man, the Palaeolithic Era gave way to the Mesolithic. The hunters of the open tundra found their hunting grounds covered with forests, which they feared and which were not suited to their methods of hunting. In the far north, tundra habitats persisted and peoples of esquimaux types continued to enjoy their traditional ways of life. On the great belts of chernozem soils, stretching from the Black Sea across Asia into North America, grasslands, prairie and steppe became developed, and the life of a nomadic hunter and later herdsman could still be pursued; such habitats were exploited by peoples of Aryan and Mongolian origin, peoples of such great vigour and resource that they continually in later times conquered the more southern peoples, effete from city dwelling, only themselves to be overthrown in time by their steppe-living relatives.

Where the forests had encroached, the Mesolithic was an era of great difficulty and tribulation. It has been most extensively studied in Scandinavian countries, especially Denmark. A fascinating first-hand account, written for the lay reader, is given by Bibby (1962a) in his book "Testimony of the Spade". In the near eastern countries, the Mesolithic lasted only a few hundred years, but was phased out progressively more slowly to the west until in Denmark it lasted at least 3000 years. This was a very long time to be regarded as transitional, and the people adapted themselves to a new way of life. They lived in differing conditions, wherever they could find a suitable niche near seashores, along rivers and far inland near lakes. The relics of human occupation have been especially studied in the Jutland Peninsula and elsewhere in Scandinavia between the inland forest and the seashore. The chief signs are great midden hillocks, composed largely of mussels and other sea shells, which show that the people were living largely on sea foods, with some forest deer and vegetable produce gleaned from the forests. The communities were not large, and in this respect conditions were similar to those in the Palaeolithic. However, the way of life and dietary habits were so drastically changed that the effect on the health of communities must have been profound. The very existence of middens is proof that potentially insanitary conditions existed favourable for the spread of enteric diseases, and life in crowded huts would favour the spread of respiratory infections. A poor survival rate is confirmed by Danish excavations north of Copenhagen from the Early Ertebølle Culture of 5000 years ago. While population numbers were too small for the development of the specific human diseases of later years, we can safely attribute the origins of many endemic disease patterns to this period. There is no evidence as to what enteric or respiratory infections became important at this time, but the confinement in restricted habitats of people with no knowledge of hygiene must have led to a serious increase of such diseases.

This difficult situation was overcome by the invention of a new form of stone tool. Whereas hitherto tools had been made by chipping or flaking flint and other suitable forms of stone, Mesolithic man initiated the new art of polishing stone, later refined to a high degree of craftsmanship in the succeeding Neolithic era. Production of polished stone axes and adzes for the first time gave man the mastery of the forests. Trees could be felled and wood could be used for useful purposes; in the Neolithic, a host of carpenter's tools were made of stone, chisels, planes and saws, comparable with those in use until recent times. Not only could forest fringes be cleared for agriculture, agricultural implements could be made and even sea-going boats.

An especially important achievement of Mesolithic peoples was the domestication of the dog from northern wolf stock. The climatic change affected wolves as well as man, and it is understandable that hungry wolves would scavenge around human settlements and some might be taken into captivity. The skills and physical attributes of wolf and man would complement each other and make it possible to hunt some of the forest animals. As a sequel, the herding skills of the now domestic dogs, half way between a husky and a German Shepherd (Alsatian), permitted the partial domestication of reindeer. In this respect too a new era in medical problems arose, because man was placed at risk or greater risk from living in close proximity to the animals he domesticated. Meanwhile, in Anatolia and other parts of the near east, man was developing a new way of life as a nomadic agriculturist. The Neolithic Era had started. An interesting account of life in Neolithic times is given by Sonia Cole in her "The Neolithic Revolution" (1965).

Disease Patterns in Neolithic Times

The Neolithic Era is divided into early and late. The late Neolithic started some 8000 years ago and gave birth to the succeeding Bronze

Age. The bronze age was a time of great prosperity with a favourable climate and world-wide trade. The scene is vividly described by Bibby (1962b) in his book "Four Thousand Years Ago". At that time, material prosperity and culture were at a higher level than in mediaeval Europe. The Neolithic Era, which led to this flowering of material comfort, started in a small way with clearance of forest or forest fringes by means of the polished stone axe. The cleared debris was burnt and seeds of barley and wheat were planted in the ashes by means of the "digging stick". Experimental attempts have been made to reproduce the conditions, one such being described by Iverson (1971). Only one or at the most two crops could be taken from the land in this way, and the nomadic agriculturists shifted slowly to new areas until, in the course of time, they had traversed the whole of Europe to the Baltic and the last traces of the Mesolithic were swept away. At the same time, cattle, sheep, goats and pigs were taken into domestication.

Meanwhile in the near east means were found whereby permanent agricultural settlements could be developed by the use of manure as fertiliser and improved agricultural implements, including a primitive plough drawn by oxen, enabled more land to be tilled more quickly. Whereas agriculture had started in hilly areas, the advantages were discovered of planting crops in flood plains, as in Mesopotamia and Egypt where the soil was renewed by silt; in time, systems of irrigation were developed as a result. Such were the beginnings of the Age of Technology, and settlements increased in size until townships were founded and from them city states. During the late Neolithic, settlements were fortified, though not during the early Neolithic. The accumulation of wealth gave incentives for robbery and war, and the need for protection.

These changes of human ecology are often called the Agricultural Revolution, but the changes were far more profound than purely agricultural. The entire social structure was altered; dietary habits were transformed; populations were increased and people came to live in crowded communities; trade routes were developed by ship and caravan to the limits of the known world; leisure and arts were able to flourish; bizarre religions appeared. The rapid change from a nomadic to a settled existence, together with unaccustomed dietary habits and the natural stresses associated with crowding, led to an unprecedented increase in the significance of infectious and other kinds of disease, which became the chief agent in controlling population levels. Not only did pre-existing disease acquire a greater significance, but new diseases, hitherto unknown, became adapted to man with dire consequences to be considered in later chapters.

CHAPTER 2

The New Diseases of Man

Civilization

The New Stone Age led imperceptibly to the age of Copper (the Chalcolithic), to the Bronze Age and thence to the Iron Age. During these times, there were four groups of peoples, who shared in the newer technologies: —
1. The Steppe-living Pastoral Nomads.
2. The Scandinavian Maritime Traders.
3. The Upland Farmers, living in fortified settlements and towns.
4. The farmers living along the great river systems, who irrigated the land.

The Steppe-living Pastoral Nomads possessed great herds of cattle and fine horses. They moved around with their herds and their families, lingering where the pasture was good. It is probable that they first made wheels and axles to carry the sledges they formerly used on the snowscape. Their chattels and their families were transported in ox-drawn tented carts. It is they who, so it seems, developed the light spoked wheel for use in horse-drawn chariots; they were, in any case skilled horsemen. In spite of their nomadic ways, they became talented metal workers making fine jewellery, horse trappings and weapons superior to those of the city dwellers to the south. They were of great courage and hardihood, and they constantly attacked and invaded the more sophisticated peoples of the towns and cities. These they burned and pillaged, but set up new urban settlements of their own; these too were in due course ravaged and occupied by new invaders from the north.

The Scandinavian peoples lived in a primitive way as small farmers. They had, however, learned to build ships and were actively engaged in trade and commerce. They sailed their ships by way of the European river systems, the well known "Amber Route" to the

Mediterranean, and over the seas along the west coast of Europe. They even formed settlements in North Africa, where their descendants still survive as the White Berbers.

The upland farmers, if we may use this term for want of a better, built their towns and cities in Asia Minor, Greece and Crete. Where their towns were situated on the great trade routes, whether overland by caravan or maritime, the merchants became very prosperous and the towns grew into cities of respectable size. Knossos and other great cities of Minoan Crete owed their existence to Crete's position as a distributive centre for trade from North Africa and Egypt on the one hand and Scandinavia on the other. Mycenae and the other Mycenean cities in Greece, including Athens, were an extension of the cultures of Anatolia and they too depended on the ports some few miles away, where ships could call.

The river based civilisations gave rise to the ancient cultures of Egypt, Mesopotamia and the Indus Valley. These people too grew prosperous by trade and commerce based on agricultural surpluses. Great cities arose, in which religion and the arts flourished, and the foundations of modern medicine were laid by two great men, Imhotep in Egypt and Asclepios in Greece. In spite of this, conditions of urbanised dwelling led to decline in cities and snail-borne disease amongst those engaged in irrigated agriculture.

Amalgamation of the city states by conquest led to the years of the great empires, the Egyptian empire, the Assyrian empire, the Persian empire, the Ptolemaic and Seleucid dynasties that arose from the conquests of Alexander, the first great native Indian empire, the Mauryan founded by Chandragupta, and so to the Roman, Spanish and British empires. Amidst pride, splendour and magnificence, conditions of unbelievable squalor existed in the growing cities, which persisted until the middle of the nineteenth century in Britain and still exist in many eastern cities to this day. The average expectation of life amongst the upper classes was no more than 40 or 50 years; amongst the lower classes, it was no more than 30. Deaths were due to accidents of childbirth both to mother and child, and to endemic, epidemic and pandemic infections. In spite of this situation, live births tended to exceed deaths and populations slowly increased so that the towns were crowded with malnourished, disease-ridden people, amongst whom an entirely new disease pattern emerged. Not only was there exacerbation of man's natural pathogens, but new diseases hitherto unknown appeared, which were virtually uncontrolled until the present century. These diseases were density-dependent, host specific to man in many cases and evidently arose by the adaptation of animal pathogens to man; indeed, some are still in the course of adaptation. While many are not zoonoses today, they originated as such.

The Diseases of Civilization

The concept that the host-specific, density-dependent diseases of civilized man were new diseases has been suggested by such workers as Aidan Cockburn (1963) in his book "The Evolution and Eradication of Infectious Disease" and by the well known Australian virologist Frank Fenner (1971) in an important paper "Infectious Disease and Social Change". Furthermore, recent researches on influenza, reviewed in the next chapter, as summarised by Beveridge (1977), have revealed the virtual certainty that the influenzas are new diseases of man, derived from animals. Density dependent diseases are those, which cause acute infection followed, if death does not intervene, by elimination of the pathogen and immunity to further attack. They tend to come in waves or epidemics sweeping through the population, then smouldering on or disappearing, until there are again enough susceptible members of the population to support a further epidemic. For these reasons, a certain minimum density of population is necessary for the survival of the pathogen which will otherwise disappear provided that there is no animal reservoir in which it can be maintained. As an example of such a disease, we shall first study measles, which is host specific to man, density dependent, and evidently had its origins in the remote past from one of man's domestic animals, the dog.

Measles

Frank Fenner (1971), on the basis of the incubation period and the period of transmissibility of measles, calculated that it could not persist in a community unless an average of 3000 cases a year should occur and that this would require a population of around 300 000. Since populations of this size did not exist until at least 6000 years ago, measles must have arisen as a new disease since then. This conclusion receives confirmation, because measles was unknown in non-urbanised populations of the world until they came in contact with city-dwelling peoples. In islands with populations of less than 500 000, the disease disappears unless reintroduced, as shown by Table 3 from Black (1966). The higher incidence of measles in Guam and Bermuda is explained by the large number of military and civilian visitors to the islands.

Measles is caused by a pseudo-myxovirus (see Chapter 3), belonging to the group described by Andrewes (1964) as the Measles-Distemper-Rinderpest Triad, three viruses which are closely related and have common antigens. Those people, who have suffered from measles, possess distemper-neutralizing antibodies in their sera. Measles virus

TABLE 3

Endemicity of measles in islands with populations of 500 000 or less, all of which had at least four exposures to measles during 1949-1964

Island	Population	Annual Pop. Input	Percentage months with measles (1949-1964)
Hawaii	550 000	16 700	100
Fiji	346 000	13 400	64
Samoa	118 000	4 400	28
Solomon	110 000	4 060	32
French Polynesia	75 000	2 690	8
Guam	63 000	2 200	80
Tonga	57 000	2 040	12
Bermuda	41 000	1 130	51
Gilbert and Ellice	40 000	1 260	15
Cook	16 000	678	6
Falkland	2 500	43	0

Black, F. L. (1966). *J. theoret. Biol.* 11, 207.

produces some immunity to distemper in ferrets. In dogs, it produces only small amounts of antibody to distemper but they show resistance to distemper on challenge; dogs recovered from distemper show antibodies to measles. In cattle, the sera of rinderpest immune animals have some neutralising power against measles, and antibodies against rinderpest may develop during the course of measles in human cases. Again rinderpest virus has immunising properties against distemper in dogs and ferrets, and rinderpest sera neutralize distemper virus. Rinderpest is so virulent in cattle as to suggest that this too is a new disease, and there appear to be no wildlife reservoirs. There can be no reasonable doubt, therefore, that both measles and rinderpest have evolved in man and cattle by mutation of distemper virus acquired originally from dogs, which inherited it from the ancestral wolves.

Distemper causes epidemics in wolves living in wild conditions, especially at times of population stress — *vide* UFAW (1976); it can also infect ferrets, and wild Mustelidae may constitute a wildlife reservoir. The reasons why distemper can maintain itself in scanty wild wolf populations, whereas measles cannot survive without a high density of human beings, appear to be threefold: — first, a reservoir may exist in wild Mustelidae; secondly, the number of generations and therefore the turnover of susceptible animals is much greater in wolves than in man; the third factor lies in the life history of wolves, which follow their prey during the winter in large numbers thus giving the opportunity for the spread of infection.

Respiratory Syncytial Virus

Cold-like symptoms are sometimes caused in man by another pseudo-myxovirus, Respiratory Syncytial Virus (R.S.V.). This virus is known as a pathogen of chimpanzees, in which it may be commensal. It is not a normal pathogen of man, in whom symptoms of the common cold are usually caused by Rhinoviruses of the Picornavirus group. The natural history of these viruses shows an interesting parallel with that of the measles virus.

The Rhinoviruses

There are some eighty distinct serotypes of human rhinoviruses, which can cause the common cold. Since immunity to all of them is impossible to acquire, epidemics of colds recur during the winter months of most years. Frank Fenner (1971) shows that, as with measles, rhinoviruses are density dependent; they do not recur in small isolated communities and do not affect persons, such as arctic explorers, who are temporarily cut off from civilization. The human rhinoviruses are host specific and could not have persisted in human communities before the days of urbanization, it is, therefore, another instance of a new disease of man, the origins of which must be sought in the mutation of an animal pathogen by which it became adapted to the human host. The only natural animal hosts of rhinoviruses are horses, so that the human rhinoviruses most probably arose from man's association with them.

As with canine distemper in wolves, the natural history of horses under wild conditions would have favoured the persistence of density dependent infections. They lived in herds, consisting of a single stallion with 30 to 50 mares, together with the young colts and fillies. Each herd had its own territory based on a water source, each territory was surrounded by the territories of other stallions and their herds. The herds, if frightened, tended to stampede, hundreds of horses from different herds becoming mixed in an apparently inextricable frenzy. Furthermore, each stallion would, in the course of time, drive away the colts and fillies of his own breeding. The colts would attempt to steal mares and form a herd of their own, failing which they would be driven from the horse ranges or killed. The fillies would have been absorbed into other herds as breeding stock. There was thus constant communication between horse herds, which may have involved many thousands of horses over large areas of territory, in days gone by, indeed, from the Black Sea to Outer Mongolia. With the extinction of horses as wild animals, such conditions plainly do not exist today, but equine rhinoviruses still persist, being spread at gymkhanas and race meetings and such functions. It is recorded by e.g. Andrewes (1964) that, when horses in a stable suffer from rhinovirus infections, grooms and stable lads may acquire infection from them, but cold epidemics are not spread from them widely in the local community. Human volunteers also become infected with typical cold symptoms from equine rhinoviruses.

The evidence suggests that there exist two host specific, new, density dependent, human, respiratory pathogens, the origins of which can be traced to animals which man has domesticated. The situation with regard to the influenzas is in some ways similar but of greater complexity. The influenzas are so important that they are dealt with at length in the next chapter. Meanwhile, attention must be paid to man's enteric infections.

Enteric Infections

Population densities, in so far as they contribute to general squalor, lack of hygiene, overcrowding and contamination of food and water, contribute materially to the incidence and severity of enteric infections. As a result of such conditions, at least three bacterial diseases have made their appearance, which are specific to man alone, though originally derived by mutation from animal sources or from organisms shared with animals. These are *Salmonella typhosa*, *Shigella dysenteriae* and *Vibrio cholerae*.

The Salmonelloses. The salmonelloses are widespread in nature and cause disease in virtually all groups of warmblooded animals. Man himself is susceptible to a wide range of salmonelloses, but only typhoid is specific to man alone; only typhoid causes such an acute and often fatal disease; its very virulence is suggestive of a new disease, in which neither host nor pathogen have become adapted to each other. *S. typhosa* may well have originated from a rodent or avian salmonella, possibly *S. typhimurium* which affects a wide range of species, especially rodents and birds. More detailed reference will be made to the salmonelloses and other enteric infections in later chapters.

The Shigelloses. The shigellae, like the salmonellae, have produced one host specific human pathogen, *Shigella dysenteriae*, of great virulence and often fatal. Man is also susceptible to other shigellae, namely those of the *S. flexneri* group, *S. sonnei* and *S. schmidtii*. The host range of the shigellae is much more restricted than that of the salmonellae and in spite of a few reports of infection in ungulates, for example Dudgeon and Urquhart (1919), Fiennes (1940), shigellae do not normally infect herbivorous animals or rodents; nevertheless, on one occasion I isolated *S. flexneri* from a porcupine at the London Zoo. The chief wild hosts of shigellae, other than *S. dysenteriae*, are apes and monkeys, *vide* Fiennes, *et al.* (1972). Such animals frequently become carriers, when it may be difficult to isolate the organisms in faecal cultures; infected monkeys constitute a serious danger to persons who come in contact with them, especially children; a number of children have died from such contacts, Fiennes (1967). *S. dysenteriae* has evidently become adapted to man as the sole host from some other shigella, probably *S. flexneri* from monkeys raiding crops or living in proximity to human habitations like the "temple" monkeys of India.

Cholera. Cholera is another enteric infection, of which man is the sole host. It was unknown outside Asia before 1817 when it appeared in Calcutta and then spread around the world. Its rapid spread was associated with insanitary conditions in towns and cities and contamination of drinking water. It may have existed in Bengal at an earlier date *vide* Pollitzer (1959), but there are no authentic records and it has probably been widely confused with bacillary dysentery in days before there were laboratory aids to diagnosis. The natural history of cholera has been reviewed by Cockburn (1963) in his book "The Evolution and Eradication of Infectious Diseases". Cockburn, in disagreement with Pollitzer, classes cholera as a "very new disease of man", which first appeared in Bengal or some neighbouring part of India and was maintained in the surface water "tanks" or ponds, which are still the main water supply of the people. He points out that there are in these waters a number of free-living *Vibrio spp.* which could by mutation and selection have become adapted to life in the human gut; he also states that a number of apparently healthy persons in such areas carry unidentified species of *Vibrio*, which could be the intermediate stage. He draws attention also to the presence of vibrios resembling *V. cholerae* in waters in many parts of the world and that they are frequent in marine and river animals. Indeed, Bengali physicians have a theory that cholera is brought up the Ganges in dry weather by a certain kind of fish. Reference to cases of enteric infection from consumption of *V. parahaemolyticus* in marine foods will be found in Chapter 13.

The theory that formerly free-living organisms become converted to pathogens seems improbable, and the conversion of an aquatic pathogen is more likely. One may also consider the possibility of mutation of an already pathogenic organism acquired from one of man's domestic animals. The obvious candidate is *V. foetus*, which is a cause of abortion in sheep and cows and has been isolated from aborted foetuses of wild living antelopes. The same organism causes acute enteritis in young pigs. More than thirty cases of *V. foetus* infection have been recorded in man, in which the symptoms are recurrent fever and lesions of the pulmonary system and digestive tract. The position of *V. foetus* as a zoonosis is reviewed by van der Hoeden (1964).

Pollitzer (1959), unlike Cockburn, finds evidence of the existence of cholera as a local endemic infection in descriptions in ancient Indian literature, though he agrees with Cockburn that the disease never became of global significance before 1817. He traces six pandemics, all of which had their origins in Bengal and spread over the world from Europe to the Americas. The first was the pandemic of 1817; the second occurred in 1829; the third in 1852; the fourth in 1863; the fifth in 1881; and the sixth in 1899. In spite of the great authority of Pollitzer, a lifelong student of cholera and the author of a long and scholarly work on the subject commissioned by WHO, Cockburn's view would seem to prevail. For our purposes, the controversy is somewhat academic. As a disease of global significance, cholera evidently did not exist before 1817 and then appeared in a series of waves or pandemics until the purification of water supplies was effected.

Venereal Diseases

Both gonorrhoea and syphilis are new diseases of man and density dependent in the sense that their spread is associated with crowded conditions and sexual promiscuity. To see how a venereal disease could be derived from animal sources is more difficult, though some rare human beings have in the past, and do still, indulge in bestial practices. However, the story of syphilis is highly intriguing and has been the subject of careful and able research, which reveals its origins as a venereal disease and suggests an animal source in the remote past. Hence our account of the venereal diseases will be confined to a study of syphilis, a disease which has been of great importance in human history. Its origins are discussed at length by Wells (1964), who shows that the disease was described in Europe at least as early as the eleventh century; he thereby disposes of the myth that it was brought to Europe by Columbus' sailors returning from the Americas. Both syphilis, caused by *Treponema pallidum*, and its parent disease yaws, caused by the allied *T. pertenue*, reveal distinctive lesions of the bones from which diagnoses can be made even in fossil material.

Researches by a French scientist André Fribourg-Blanc (1972) have recently revealed that a treponematosis exists in African monkeys. The disease causes mild skin lesions and swelling of the regional lymph glands; it can be detected serologically and the treponeme can be isolated in culture. The disease closely resembles the human treponematosis known as "pinta", which occurs in South America, except that pinta is more severe than the monkey disease and tends to recur throughout life. In neither disease are there deep lesions, nor is the skeleton ever affected. In South America, the infection is endemic but wild living primates are not affected; no animals other than man and chimpanzees have been infected experimentally. Clearly, there exist closely related treponemes which infect man in South America and monkeys in Africa; the hosts are well adapted and the diseases of no great significance. It is tempting to propose a common origin of the diseases in the remote past.

In Africa, human populations suffer from no mild endemic diseases resembling pinta or the monkey treponematosis. However, in areas of the wet tropics, where monkeys are affected, human populations suffer from endemic yaws. This a serious disease, which affects the liver and other internal organs and causes characteristic lesions of the skeleton. The probable course of events has been suggested by Hackett (1975), formerly adviser on treponematoses to the World Health Organization. Hackett shows that there exists another human treponematosis known as "treponarid" or "endemic syphilis", although it is not a venereal disease. Treponarid is endemic in human populations in the dry tropics, in contrast to yaws which is only found in the wet tropics; its range extends through the dry tropics north through India to northern Siberia and south to central Australia. In Africa, the Kalahari Bushmen are infected with it; in Pakistan, India, Ceylon, Indonesia and New Guinea, it is associated only with populations of Stone Age peoples of Australoid type; peoples of other racial groups are not affected.

Endemic syphilis is thus associated with peoples in a primitive stage of culture, who wear little or no clothing and whose way of life is largely nomadic; therefore, it is not a density dependent form of disease. According to Hackett (personal communication), the Aborigines entered Australia in four waves of immigration between 30 000 and 18 000 B.C., after which the level of the sea rose and they were isolated; see also Mulvaney (1966) and Macintosh (1967). There is no evidence of endemic syphilis in people of the first two waves, who eventually occupied lands in Tasmania and South Australia. The third wave settled in Central Australia and the fourth in the north. At any one time, 2% of these populations are infected with endemic syphilis. The northern Aborigines have had occasional contact with Indonesians washed up in their canoes and the disease could conceivably have been introduced in this way; this is, however, unlikely, because Indonesian peoples are not naturally infected with treponarid, and the separation of the northern from the central Aborigines has been so complete. This new disease must, therefore, have appeared in Stone Age peoples between, say, 25 000 B.C. and 18 000 B.C. We thus have a trail of disease evolution, which may well be: — Monkey treponematosis - - - ► Pinta (S. America) - - - ► Yaws(Africa, wet tropics) - - - ► Endemic

Syphilis (Africa, dry tropics). The disease then shows a trail of migration from the Bushmen, who at one time were widespread over the whole of Africa, to Pakistan, where Australoid people were present at the time of the Indus Valley civilization, to Australoid settlements in India, Ceylon and Indonesia, and thence to Australia.

Venereal syphilis was undoubtedly evolved from endemic syphilis under crowded urbanised conditions. The change from contact infection to venereal, as suggested by Hackett (1975), was the result of the wearing of clothes so that skin to skin intimacy only occurred regularly during copulation. Just when and where venereal syphilis first appeared has not yet been determined and there is little reliable evidence either from fossil material or from the imprecise accounts of disease symptoms from early times. Both Wells (1964) and Hackett (personal communication) attach importance to accounts of the use of mercurial ointments in treatment of diseases, sometimes described as leprosy, because they point out that mercury would be ineffective against any disease other than syphilis. For this reason, Hackett postulates that syphilis had made its appearance by Graeco-Roman times, when the use of mercury for treatment of disease was widespread.

It would serve little purpose to trace the origins of other venereal diseases. The *Neisseria* of gonorrhoea is no doubt a urino-genital variant of that which is commensal in human throats and allied to *N. meningitidis*. *Herpes simplex* type 2 virus is similarly a urino-genital variant of *H. simplex* type 1; its possible role in the etiology of cervical carcinoma of women and of prostatic cancers in men is discussed in Chapter 4. Meanwhile, as a sequel to syphilis, we may pass to two of the most important new diseases of man, both of which can cause lesions of the skeleton as can yaws and syphilis, namely leprosy and tuberculosis.

Leprosy and Tuberculosis

Leprosy and tuberculosis are the two important diseases of man, which are caused by acid fast bacilli, the one by *Mycobacterium leprae*, the other by *Mycobacterium tuberculosis*. Of the latter, there are two important strains, *M.t. hominis* and *M.t. bovis*; though only classified as strains, the distinction is of great importance in human disease ecology. Both leprosy and tuberculosis, at any rate that caused by *M.t. hominis*, are new diseases of man, their survival being dependent on squalor and crowding. The ecology of the two diseases is of especial interest, because they appear to be mutually exclusive. *M. leprae* and *M.t. hominis* are related acid fast bacilli and create some degree of cross-immunity. Thus in Japan, as shown by Yanasigawa (1958), BCG vaccine used in the control of tuberculosis protected the children of leprous mothers from leprosy. Cockburn (1963) suggested that tuberculosis of the human type appeared as a new disease during the Middle Ages, before which the chief disease caused by acid fast bacilli was leprosy. In Scandinavia, according to Moller-Christensen (1961), leprosy was common before the twelfth century but no cases of tuberculosis of the skeleton have been found. In his excavations of the mediaeval leper cemetery at Aaderup in Denmark, he found over two hundred cases, which could be positively diagnosed. Since this was only one of many leprosaria in the country, the disease must have been very common. In England, according to Wells (1964), there were some two hundred leper hospitals in the thirteenth century and, as in other parts of Europe, the disease was widespread; however, within a few hundred years leprosy had vanished and tuberculosis was widespread.

Traditionally, leprosy is associated in people's minds with the Holy Land. However, there is little positive evidence to support this and Wells (1964) points to uncertainties of diagnosis in early times, by which both syphilis and a great many diseases of the skin were classified as leprosy. Nevertheless, leprosy does seem to have posed problems during the Exodus, and detailed rules of diagnosis and quarantine are prescribed under Mosaic Law, as recorded in Leviticus 13. The subject is reviewed in my earlier book "Man, Nature and Disease", Fiennes (1964). Leprosy appears to have originated in the Far East, and reliable references to its existence appear in Indian literature as early as 600 B.C., and even its treatment by chaulmoogra oil, which is still used. There is no disease which is less readily transmitted from patient to patient than leprosy, or so easily controlled by simple methods of hygiene or by what we should today regard as normal standards of cleanliness. Persons working in leper settlements rarely contract the disease unless rules of hygiene are neglected, and even in the case of spouses of lepers the infection rate is below 10%. Infection usually arises from prolonged and intimate contact between persons, particularly between a mother and her child. The disease is not, however, congenital and children are never born infected. Sometimes infection contracted in childhood does not show itself until the twentieth year or later. It is, thus, a disease of insidious nature, associated with poor conditions of life, poverty and dirt.

It cannot be said with certainty that leprosy could not have existed in stone age times as with the density dependent infections. That it should have done so is, however, most improbable. No evidence of it has been found in fossil material, and any small nomadic band in which it appeared would surely not be able to survive the rigours of the climate and the way of life. *M. leprae* is, however, species specific for man and there are few wildlife sources from which infection could have originated. As stated, the evidence suggests that the disease originated in the Far East, and it is here that the most probable source of infection is to be found in the water buffalo. In many Far Eastern countries, water buffaloes are the most important of the domestic animals, providing most of the milk and meat, while cattle are used as working animals. In some countries, such as Malaya, a form of skin leprosy is very common in them; sectioned lesions stained for acid fast bacilli show them to be packed with organisms. It is most probable that human leprosy originated from contact with these animals, or with their skins used as sleeping mats or clothing.

As already stated, there is no evidence for the existence of the human type of tuberculosis before the late Middle Ages, when it replaced leprosy. It then emerges as a new, density dependent, specifically human disease. There can be little doubt that it originated from a mutation of the bovine bacillus. Tuberculosis is discussed at greater length in a later chapter, and we can now examine its probable origins. Bovine tuberculosis is evidently of much greater antiquity than human. According to Wells (1964), there is dubious evidence of bovine tuberculosis in Neolithic skeletons. However, it was evidently widespread in Ancient Egypt as revealed both by actual diagnoses in mummified bodies, and by numerous pictorial representations of Pott's Disease or tuberculosis of the spine. It is to be recalled that lesions of the skeleton are characteristic of bovine tuberculosis and are only rarely found with human. In many representations of cattle also, the animals have the appearance of advanced tuberculosis, and Wells (1964) draws attention to a bas-relief from Mer XII dynasty, in which both cattle and herdsman appear to be in an advanced stage of the disease. Infection would be acquired from milk and meat from infected cattle. Bovine tuberculosis, therefore, qualifies as a new disease of man acquired from one of his domestic animals, the human type of disease arising from the bovine at a later date. The ancestral wild cattle were no doubt sporadically infected, the disease becoming serious under conditions of domestication.

Diphtheria

Another serious disease of civilized man, which also has a connection with milk, is diphtheria, of which the origins are somewhat mysterious. The causal organism, *Corynebacterium diphtheriae* occurs in two forms; one produces toxin, the other does not. The first description of it is given by a medical writer of the sixth century A.D., Aretaeus of Cappadocia. It then reappears in sixteenth century Spain under the name of "garotillo". Since those days, diphtheria developed into one of the most deadly and tragic diseases of children affecting chiefly the 5-10 age group with a death rate up to 10%. It plainly qualifies as a new disease of man and up to a point is density dependent. However, it was prevalent in country districts as well as towns, and my research into a parish register a few years ago revealed a high death rate in the 5-10 age group most likely due to diphtheria. An animal host of *C. diphtheriae* is the cow, which suffers from mild ulceration of the udder and transmits the disease in the milk thus accounting for the high incidence in country children. Transmission by milk was first described by Dean and Todd (1902) — quoted by Wilson amd Miles (1953).

As a virulent pathogen *C. diphtheriae* affects man alone, but there are odd records of the organism being isolated on rare occasions from other animals, such as horses (Minett, 1920), cats (Simmons, 1920), fowls (Litterer, 1925) — references all quoted by Wilson and Miles (1953). It is impossible even to guess at the origins of *C. diphtheriae*. A number of corynebacteria are found in animals, both as harmless commensals and as pathogens (for example *C. ovis* in sheep). Commensal corynebacteria may be isolated also from the throats of healthy humans; one evidently at some time developed the power to manufacture toxin and some people became carriers of *C. diphtheriae*. As a result of the widespread use of vaccines, the disease has today virtually disappeared.

Other New Diseases

Typhus is one of the best examples of a new disease, because the intermediate stage, murine typhus, still exists as well as the host specific classical typhus; it is considered in detail in Chapter 8. Plague, though of ancient lineage in its sylvatic and perhaps in its bubonic form, qualifies as a new disease of animal origin in its pneumonic form. Smallpox can undoubtedly be classed as a new disease of man, density dependent and originating as a zoonosis, possibly from a mutation of the cowpox virus.

There are a great many other viruses, to which the human race is prey, belonging to many different groups. Some may be new diseases; some may not. Some may still await discovery. A virus, which for long defied discovery, was that of Infectious Hepatitis, one of the Enterovirus group. Whereas this disease appears to be chiefly endemic in character, it shows some disturbing features. Both chimpanzees and some monkey species suffer from inapparent infection, though serological tests show that there is subclinical liver damage. Consequently, persons who handle primates in laboratories and elsewhere are at greater risk than the rest of the population. A further danger from this virus arises from the increasing pollution of estuary and inland waters which can serve as a vehicle for its transmission. If not a new disease of man — and it may well be one — it has given rise to a new disease in very recent times, that of Serum Hepatitis, from which it can be distinguished serologically. Serum hepatitis is a mutant of infectious hepatitis; its chief characteristic lies in its mode of transmission, which occurs solely by artificial means from the injection of vaccines containing serum from persons carrying the virus. In this it resembles Vaccinia, the mutated smallpox virus used for vaccination; this virus too can only be spread by deliberate human agency.

Poliomyelitis presents a peculiar anomaly of human disease ecology, which deserves brief mention. Poliovirus is the best known of the enteroviruses and would appear to be a normal commensal of the human gut, provided that infection is acquired in early infancy. In older children the virus becomes invasive and may attack the nervous system. Thus, the virus is only dangerous, when standards of nursery hygiene are high; children reared in dirty conditions do not suffer from paralytic poliomyelitis. Other enteroviruses, such as the Coxsackie and Echovirus sub-groups, sometimes cause symptoms similar to poliomyelitis in human beings. As a zoonosis, there is a single report of the disease being transmitted to a child by a budgerigar. A serious naturally occurring outbreak of poliomyelitis in apes was reported by Allmond *et al.* (1967). Paralytic disease due to poliovirus type 1 was observed in a captive orang utan and two gorillas; additionally, two gorillas, nine orang utans, twelve chimpanzees and three monkeys were found to be excreting type 1 poliovirus. Heberling (1972) reporting on routine virus isolates from imported monkeys found three of seventy six such isolates to be poliovirus type 3, together with 41 coxsackie viruses. It is sometimes said that poliomyelitis is not a zoonosis; however, it would be unwise for non-immunised personnel to handle imported primates.

One could pursue the speculation as to the evolution of diseases, which attack urbanised and industrial man almost endlessly. It should, however, be apparent from what has been written to what an extent the disease pattern has changed since Stone Age times. Population numbers are no longer controlled by natural ecological factors; birth rates have been high during historical times and the death rate has been high also for the most part due to acute and chronic disease. Many diseases, which have taken such a toll of human life are new diseases; many have originated as zoonoses from animal sources, but have become so adapted to man that they infect him only to the exclusion of all other animal species. Evidently, new disease patterns are still evolving and new crises may still emerge; some of the older diseases are acquiring new significance from recent changes in our way of life.

CHAPTER 3

Pandemic Diseases

The Characteristics of Pandemic Disease Outbreaks

A pathogen, capable of spreading global pandemics, must possess certain rather special characteristics: —

1. It must be capable of rapid transmission from one host to another.

2. It must find susceptible hosts in sufficient numbers to sustain its momentum.

3. To fulfil the first criterion, it virtually must be spread by airborne infection. This limits the power to cause global pandemics to respiratory pathogens, plague, for example, does not become pandemic until the pneumonic form develops from the bubonic.

It is probably because of these restrictions that only two diseases have so far spread across the whole world in pandemic fashion, plague and influenza. The two pathogens overcome the problem of finding susceptible subjects in different ways. In man, immunity to plague is short-lived. With influenza, the immunity is more durable but the virus exists in different guises, being capable of changing its antigenic structure, so that new or differing strains continually appear.

Epidemic diseases recur at intervals in populations, which have had previous experience of them so that only a proportion, usually the young and the old, are susceptible; pandemics are new diseases or new sub-types of diseases, to which the population has no resistance whatever. The distinction is clearly seen in influenza, in which epidemics of the same sub-type appear at three to four yearly intervals, and new antigenic sub-types appear every thirty to forty years. Local disease pandemics, caused by diseases introduced from different geographical areas, may have devastating effects, as has occurred in many places with yellow fever and malaria, but global spread is prevented for ecological reasons.

The Causes and Consequences of Pandemics

A great many diseases have had profound effects on the course of history, some of which will be mentioned briefly in later chapters. Recurrent plague pandemics have had a special significance, in that the most serious have always occurred at times of social stress, when population numbers have outstripped resources, either because numbers have increased unduly or because climatic deterioration has resulted in bad harvests. These problems have been discussed by a number of authors, such as Banks (1969), Bourne (1975, 1976), Dempster (1975), Eckholm (1976), Ehrlich and Ehrlich (1970), Ehrlich *et al.* (1973) and Hollingsworth (1973). The role of plague as a controller of human population levels has been so important, that a brief survey of the major pandemic outbreaks will be given under. There has been no global plague pandemic affecting western countries, since that which reached England in 1665, and it is generally believed that conditions today are such that the disease could not recur in this form. It is, however, significant that the last great pandemic of comparable importance was due to influenza. It occurred in the stricken years of 1918 to 1919, when the world was in the last agonies of the First World War.

Since 1918, there have occurred two more influenza pandemics due to the appearance of new sub-types of the virus. Neither has been accompanied by an alarmingly high death rate, and it might seem reasonable to postulate that a deterioration of living standards is necessary to convert global pandemic into global tragedy. This assumption is unfortunately too facile. Experience with myxomatosis in rabbits, with fowl plague in poultry, and even with many human diseases in isolated communities shows that pathogens can appear, which kill more than 98% of populations living in healthy hygienic conditions. Nevertheless, it is evident that poorer living standards can contribute to the toll of life during pandemics and possibly permit the antigenic change of a pathogen which must precede its pandemic spread. While only two pathogens have so far been involved in human pandemics, there is no reason to suppose that a third may not emerge in the future. An understanding of the natural history of the two so far involved is, therefore, important.

Plague

The Natural History of Plague (*vide* van der Hoeden; 1964)

It is generally believed that plague originated as an inapparent infection of gerbils in eastern Asia, being transmitted by the gerbil fleas. As a disease of man, it was endemic, sporadic cases occurring when some person was bitten by infected gerbil fleas or by fleas from rats that had acquired infection from the gerbils. At the present time, there exist endemic plague centres in many parts of the world, in which the wild rodent hosts vary greatly. In South Africa, they are the gerbils (*Tatera* and *Desmodillus*), ground squirrels (*Geosciurus*), multimammate mice (*Mastomys*) and striped mice (*Rhabdomys*). In the western states of North America, reservoirs of infection exist in ground squirrels (*Citellus*), tree squirrels (*Sciurus*), chipmunks (*Eutamias*), marmots (*Marmota*), woodrats (*Neotoma*) and prairie dogs (*Cynomys*). In South America, the wild hosts are cuis (*Cavia, Microcavia, Graomys, Galea*) and viscachas (*Lagostomus*). In the steppe lands, where plague is believed to have originated, extending from south-eastern Europe through central Asia, Mongolia, and southern Siberia to the Pacific, plague is harboured by susliks (*Citellus*), ground squirrels (*Citellus spermophilus*), the marmot known as tarabagan (*Arctomys*), jerboas (*Allactaga, Dipodipus*), gerbils (*Meriones*) and field mice (*Microtus*). In these latter areas, human populations are sparse and the people are nomadic; plague smoulders on in a sporadic way and has been called "sylvatic plague". Occasional human cases may occur, for example when a hunter traps an infected wild rodent; then, transmission is direct from the wild rodent fleas to man.

Plague cannot persist endemically in human populations, though it does so in wild rodents. Rats, which survive infection, often become "carriers" and the rat fleas survive for long periods in the nests passing infection to new generations of young rats. As a result, occasional epidemics occur among the rodents, by which their numbers are greatly reduced. It is at such times that the two species of rats whose lives are associated with man, the brown rat (*Rattus norvegicus*) and the black rat (*R. rattus*), become involved in epidemics; the black rat is more often associated with the great pandemics, possibly because it is more inclined to travel and to invade ships or because its fleas are more aggressive to man.

The fleas, which infest brown rats, are *Ceratophyllus fasciatus*; those of the black rat are *Xenopsylla cheopis, X. astia* and *X. brasiliensis. X. cheopis* is the flea usually associated with rat to man transmission of plague. Plague bacilli enter the flea's stomach with ingested blood and multiply to such an extent that the entrance to the stomach becomes obstructed. The flea leaves the dead rat and, being hungry though unable to feed, seeks another host; rat or human. In attempting to feed, some of the fresh blood contaminated with plague bacilli is regurgitated and is likely to be rubbed into the bite wound because of the irritation. Where the flea's gut is not completely obstructed, bacilli may be passed in the faeces and infect wounds or abrasions. It has been suggested that plague can also be transmitted from man to man by human fleas, *Pulex irritans*. However, there is no evidence of this, although these fleas are very common in some areas where plague epidemics still occur, such as India. It has been observed in India that the brown rats become infected first and the black rats later. This would give a disease cycle as follows: — wild rodent ---→flea ---→brown rat ----→flea ---→ black rat ---→flea ---→ man (bubonic plague) ----→man by droplet (pneumonic plague). Recovered human beings develop an immunity to reinfection, which is very transitory; in rats the immunity is durable; this explains why epidemics in rats, hence in human populations, are cyclic.

The Antiquity of Plague

There is no reason to suppose that some wild rodent populations have not been carriers of *Yersinia (Pasteurella) pastis* from time immemorial. If so, plague in its sylvatic form is a very old disease and no doubt claimed some victims among the hunters of the Old Stone Age. It is often suggested that the earliest accounts of plague outbreaks are to be found in the Old Testament. One occurred around the year 1100 B.C. and is recounted in the first book of Samuel, chapters 4 to 7. The children of Israel were defeated in battle by the Philistines, who captured the Ark of God. Subsequently, wherever the ark was sent, the Philistines suffered from some epidemic disease, characterised by "emerods" in their private parts. Upwards of fifty thousand Philistines were said to have died. If the word bubo is substituted for emerod, we have, so it is surmised, an account of plague associated with mice in coastal towns. After seven months, the ark was returned together with an offering of seven golden emerods and seven golden mice, suggesting that the Philistines associated the plague with mice.

The history of plague pandemics is reviewed by Ziegler (1969). There is no evidence that any great pandemic occurred until the years A.D. 592 to 594 in the reign of the Roman emperor Justinian, whose capital was Constantinople. The outbreak originated in Arabia, whence it reached Egypt and was spread from the trading centre of Pelusium over the whole known world. This pandemic killed about half the population of the Roman Empire, which was so weakened that it was never able to recover. It reached England and Ireland in A.D. 664, where it was known as the Plague of Cadwalader's time. Epidemic plague was certainly present in Europe from the middle of the eleventh century to the end of the sixteenth century, reaching pandemic proportions in the fourteenth century. In 1661 plague reappeared in Europe in pandemic form, and local epidemics were recurring until the middle of the eighteenth century. The last great pandemic appeared in Canton and Hongkong in 1894, whence it spread to Japan, India and Asia Minor in 1896. During the next two years, it appeared in many parts of the Far East, Australia, Mauritius, Madagascar, parts of the Middle and Near East, Portugal, Scotland and South America. It appeared in California in 1900. It is likely that the widespread endemic foci throughout the world resulted from this pandemic. In all pandemics, the pestilence was spread by way of the great maritime trade routes and the vehicles of infection were the shipboard rats and their fleas. The spread inland from the busy ports was mostly by direct man to man infection of the pneumonic form of the disease, although the insanitary conditions of towns and cities and, no doubt, the high population of rats would be a contributory factor. Experience of plague in more recent times suggests that the great pandemics of the past are unlikely to be repeated in the improved living conditions of modern times.

Both the great plague pandemic of A.D. 592-594 and the Black Death occurred at times of great social stress, and most students of the subject attribute significance to this. The appearance of plague in A.D. 592 merely hastened the end of the Roman Empire. The civilised world was being ravaged by invasions of the Goths and Visigoths from the north and by the Huns under Attila from the Russian steppes; the Vandals were overrunning North Africa. Attila was preparing to attack Latium itself, but abandoned the plan, when he learned that plague was raging in Rome. However, let us look at the history of the Black Death in greater detail for a picture of the conditions in which pandemic diseases are liable to appear.

The Black Death

Good accounts of the Black Death are given by Lange (1969) and by Ziegler (1969). The eleventh and twelfth centuries in Europe were times of great prosperity, the Golden Age of the high Middle Ages. The climate was warm and equable; agriculture was prosperous and people were well fed and living comfortably in small communities. Then the population increased beyond the capacity of agriculture to provide sufficient food and widespread starvation followed. Attempts were made to overcome the situation by industrialisation and people moved into cities, creating slums which were breeding grounds of many diseases. In central and western Europe, the land under cultivation had reached a level, which was not attained again for 500 years. In many parts, population densities were higher in A.D. 1260 than at any time until the 1950s. Towns had increased in size to ten or twenty thousand inhabitants, an unprecedented size for the time and quite unmanageable in ignorance of the principles of local government and sanitation. In rural areas too, numbers had increased greatly but the agriculture of the time could not cope with the increased numbers and additional land available for development was becoming scarce. The difficult situation was aggravated by a change of climate. The polar ice cap and glaciers moved south; the climate became colder; the growing season was shortened and the cloud cover increased. There were five grave famines in England between 1272 and 1311 and every European country lost at least one harvest between 1315 and 1319. Conditions in the years 1332, 1345 and 1348 were especially difficult. The famine conditions were intensified, because the lack of hot summer sun hindered the production of salt by evaporation of salt water and salt was in short supply for the preservation of the winter meat supplies.

The origins of the plague are believed to have been in wild rodents in the steppes of Russia, and not in endemic foci which, as we have seen, already existed in Europe. Initially, it spread eastwards into China and India. Between China and Persia, conditions, arising from climatic disasters, floods and earthquakes were as serious as in Europe, where disturbing rumours were spread of unprecedented disaster. "India was depopulated; Tartary, Mesopotamia, Syria and Armenia were covered with dead bodies; the Kurds fled in vain to the mountains. In Caramania and Caesarea none were left alive . . .". It did not occur to the peoples of Europe that their turn came next. However, when 85 000 people died in the Crimea — in those days the great entrepot for trade between east and west — Europe's fate was sealed.

From the Crimea, the disease was carried in the trading galleys, first to parts of Italy, Sicily, Venice and Genoa. It was taken by plague-stricken galleys, refused admission to Genoa, to Marseilles and thence to Spain and the Balearic Isles. Wherever the galleys went, new foci of bubonic plague were created, from which spread the pneumonic pandemic through weakened and debilitated populations. At this time, England was relatively prosperous in spite of the famine years. Agriculture was thriving and the few towns were wealthy, if insanitary. However, Edward III was squandering the national resources on unnecessary wars against France and Scotland. Bubonic plague appeared in the south and west at the end of June 1348, but it did not develop the pneumonic pandemic form until the following August. It was subsequently introduced to eastern and northern ports. By December 1349, the disease had run its course but about half the population had died. The death rate throughout Europe is variously estimated as between 40% and 60% and no doubt varied in different areas. The toll was certainly higher amongst urban communities than rural. The population of England at that time is unknown, since there had been no census since that of the Domesday Book in A.D. 1086; it is thought to have been between four and five million.

Social Consequences of the Black Death

In spite of the enormous numbers of deaths, nowhere in European cities did administration break down. Somehow the people coped. The dead were buried and measures of hygiene were put into effect. Most of the doctors and clergy performed the tasks imposed by their professions in a selfless fashion, although many died of the plague as a result of their exposure to infection. It was a tribute to the character of the people in those desperate mediaeval times. Their tribulations were largely attributed to the visitations of God for their sins, though some did question the judgement of the Almighty in dispensing justice so impartially to the just and the wicked alike. The death toll, as one would expect, was higher amongst the poor and chronically mal-nourished living in squalid conditions. The enormous loss of numbers in the labouring class led to a major social revolution, the end of the feudal system. Landlords were in difficulty; they were forced to pay higher wages although there was a reduced demand for their produce because of the smaller population, and the great estates began to be broken up. Serfs and villeins, when labour was so scarce, could demand large increases in benefits and wages and, if not granted could move elsewhere and, if they wished, go to the towns; this, though illegal, could not be prevented. In the long run, the effects of the Black Death were beneficial. The higher wages and greater mobility of labour were of advantage for the future and laid the foundations of the prosperity and vigour of the people that were to develop in Tudor times; furthermore the movements of population to towns and workshops laid the foundation for the Industrial Revolution four hundred years later. While it cannot be said that the Black Death initiated any major changes, it certainly accelerated them and hastened the end of the feudal system.

Plague continued to recur in Europe during the fourteenth, fifteenth, sixteenth and seventeenth centuries but the results were never again so serious or the mortality so high. The Great Plague of London occurred in 1665 and killed 60 000 of the city's 450 000 population; this was a serious tragedy, but not to an extent which disrupted life greatly. In the Far East, outbreaks of plague continued into the twentieth century, Between 1898 and 1918, ten million deaths occurred in the city of Bombay alone.

There are many lessons to be learned from the story of plague, an insignificant pasteurellosis of obscure rodents living in a remote and inaccessible part of the world. Before assessing the importance of pandemics, the situation must be studied in relation to influenza both as a global pathogen causing pandemics and as a zoonosis.

Influenza — the Myxoviruses

Table 4 gives a classification of the myxovirus group, to which the influenza viruses belong.

The myxoviruses belong to the RNA group of viruses. The virion consists of a protein core containing eight genes and a protein coat or "capsid" within a plasma membrane of lipoprotein. The core contains

TABLE 4
Classification of myxovirus groups

Virus Group	Common Name	Natural Hosts and Susceptibles
Myxovirus	Influenza A	Man, swine, horse, wild and domestic birds
	Influenza B	Man
	Influenza C	Man
	Influenza D	Man, pig, mice (Japan only)
	Fowl Plague	Domestic fowl
	Other bird viruses	Wild and domestic birds
Paramyxovirus	Parainfluenza 1	Man, mouse
	Parainfluenza 2	Man
	Parainfluenza 3	Man, cattle
	Parainfluenza 4	Man
	Parainfluenza 5	Man, monkey
	Mumps	Man
	Newcastle disease	Birds, man
Pseudomyxovirus	Foamy viruses	Monkeys, chimpanzees
	Respiratory syncytial virus	Chimpanzees, man
	Distemper	Dog
	Rinderpest	Cattle
	Measles	Man

the genetic information for replication and construction of proteins, including enzymes. The capsid possesses the two important enzymes, which determine infectivity and cell penetration; these are haemagglutinin (H) and neuraminidase (N). Both enzymes are strongly antigenic and immunity to myxovirus infection is dependent on possession of neutralising antibody to both. The core antigens are believed to be group specific (gs), but the arrangement and types of H and N antigens determine the species specificity and sub-type of the virus. During the course of replication, the eight genes become separated with an important result, namely that, if more than one sub-type of virus is present in a single cell, hybridised or "recombinant" virions may emerge carrying hybrid genetic information. The implications are considered under.

Types B, C and D myxoviruses have a limited host range and tend to recur in mild epidemic form. The great pandemics are associated with myxovirus A infections with changed H and N antigen combinations. It is worthy of note that the true myxoviruses are not natural pathogens of primates other than man.

The Natural History of Influenza

An excellent review of influenza is given by Burnet (1962). However, his account has been overtaken by events, and the latest information is succinctly given by Beveridge (1977) in his "Influenza: The Last Great Plague". Epidemics of influenza show certain characteristic features, which serve to identify them from historical records. The earliest record from English history, according to Burnet (1962), is of an outbreak occurring in A.D. 1170, and there have been recurring incidents since then. However, certainly until the time of Louis XIV of France influenza was not regarded as a serious disease and it was something of a joke when the courtiers one by one began to sneeze and splutter. Possibly these outbreaks were not due to Group A virus.

Beveridge (1977) has been at great pains to assess what historical outbreaks could be considered as pandemics as opposed to epidemics. The following assessment is abridged from his book: —

1729-30 (probably pandemic). Influenza widespread in Europe; high attack rate, appreciable mortality. In London regarded as a new disease. Only 1% escaped infection. During September, 1000 deaths per week.

1732-33 (pandemic). Influenza worldwide. In Plymouth, England, some were seized suddenly, "they fell down in multitudes, scarce anyone escaped it". Probably started in Moscow, though some say Connecticut.

1742-43 (probably pandemic). Influenza widespread in Europe. In Rome, 80 000 ill; 500 buried in one day. In London, the death rate trebled at the beginning of April.

1761-62 (probably pandemic). N. America and W. Indies affected in 1761; Europe 1762. Mortality variable; very high in Breslau in February 1762.

1767 (probably pandemic). Influenza reported in all N. America and most of Europe. Unimportant in Britain.

1775-76 (probably pandemic). All Europe and the Near and Far East affected. Little mortality in England.

1781-82 (pandemic). This was a devastating pandemic affecting all European countries, China, India and N. America; one of the most widespread that has ever occurred. Both incidence and death rate very high. The pandemic was at its height during the summer months, strong evidence that it was a true pandemic. Started in China during the autumn.

1800-02 (pandemic). A mild form of the disease, which spread over all Europe, China and Brazil. Started in Russia or China.

1830-33 (pandemic). Influenza diffused over the whole world in the course of three years. In Britain, it started in the early summer of 1831 and became really serious in 1833; overall death rate quadrupled in London during the worst two weeks. The pandemic started in China in January.

1847-48 (pandemic). Influenza widespread in Europe, N. America, W. Indies and Brazil. High incidence and high mortality. More deaths in London than from the cholera epidemic of 1832. Probably started in Russia in March.

1889-90 (pandemic). There were doubtful pandemics in 1857-58 and 1873-75, which had a peculiar distribution in that Britain was virtually spared. In 1889 there occurred the so-called Asiatic influenza pandemic, which started in Bukhara in Russia in May. The pandemic spread slowly at first, but covered the entire world with a high attack rate and heavy mortality.

Influenza; the Pandemics of 1918-19 and After

The terrible pandemic of so-called Spanish Flu swept the entire world from 1918-19; the toll of deaths was 3-5 per thousand of the entire world population with total deaths between 15 and 25 million. In England alone 150 000 people died. During its course, some unusual features were revealed. Deaths were much higher in persons of non-European origin than in Europeans. For example the death rate in South Africans of Bantu origin was 27 per thousand; in India, from 4 to 60 per thousand died, with total deaths reaching five million. In Samoa, 25% of the population died. The pandemic occurred in three waves in less than twelve months. The first wave appeared in the spring of 1918; the disease was mild and mortality not unusually high. Those affected were mostly young adults. The second wave came in the autumn of 1918, causing a very high mortality; 50% of cases were in the 20-40 age group, a most unusual feature. The third wave early in 1919 was less severe.

After 1919, epidemics of influenza recurred at irregular intervals due to the same sub-type of virus, until 1957 when it was superseded by another sub-type and a new pandemic known as Asian Flu. Asian flu started in China in February and reached Europe and the Americas in June. The disease caused some 60 000 deaths in the United States between October 1957 and March 1958, mostly in persons over 65 years of age. However, the attack rate was highest in the 10-20 age group.

In 1968, a new pandemic started in south east China in July known as Hongkong Flu. In the USA, some 80 000 deaths resulted. In Europe, there were very few deaths during the first winter, but during the next winter (1969-70) the disease recurred with greater severity with 30 000 deaths in an eight week period in Britain alone; these occurred mostly in older age groups.

It is regarded as axiomatic by students of influenza (*vide* Beveridge, 1977) that each new antigenic sub-type of influenza A displaces the previous one. Thus Spanish flu continued to appear every few years in epidemic form, until displaced by Asian flu; the same occurred with Asian flu until it was displaced by Hongkong. No two sub-types coexist at the same time. Nevertheless, it appears that former sub-types can reappear, for example the 1889 sub-type is believed to have been the same as Hongkong as judged by serological tests on stored blood sera of elderly people. At the present time (February 1978), an unusual situation appears to have arisen in that the variant of Spanish Flu, which was prevalent between 1940 and 1957, the so-called Red Flu, has reappeared while the Hongkong sub-type is still active.

Influenza as a Zoonosis

An American veterinary surgeon, Richard Shope (1931, 1936, 1943, 1955), in a series of classical experiments demonstrated the identity of Swine Influenza virus in Iowa with the human virus of the 1918-19 pandemic. In the pigs, the virus had become neither epidemic nor pandemic, but endemic involving a major change in the relationships of the virus with its host. Shope found the virus to be resident in pig lungworms from which it did not emerge to cause influenza, unless the pig suffered from respiratory disease due to the bacterium *Haemophilus suis*, or was subjected to some form of stress. The lungworm is responsible for carrying the virus from pig to pig, for which it requires an intermediate host, this being an earthworm; the pig eats the earthworm and the lungworm develops in the pig's lungs. More recent studies have shown that today the virus has become better adapted to the pig and direct pig to pig infection occurs. The virus has become endemic in the pig; the adults harbour the virus from one year to the next and the young pigs become infected after weaning.

The virus of swine influenza retained the surface antigens of Spanish Flu virus but apparently lost the power to reinfect human hosts. Until 1976, only one case of influenza of this sub-type was reported in a human being; this was in a boy suffering from Hodgkin's Disease and under treatment for it; both the disease and the treatment would render him more susceptible. However, in January 1976 an epidemic of swine influenza occurred in an American army camp at Fort Dix, New Jersey, causing one death in some eighteen cases. So alarmed was the American government that one million dollars was spent on preparing vaccine against the possibility of a new pandemic. The swine virus was in competition with the current epidemic strain of Hongkong virus, which proved the more aggressive, and the swine virus disappeared.

Swine, equine, avian and human viruses rarely cross the species barrier. The exception to this rule lies with the current Hongkong virus, which has caused widespread outbreaks of influenza in pigs in China and Czecho-Slovakia. It was also experimentally transmitted to Bonnet Macaque monkeys (*Macaca radiata*) and spread naturally among them, a most unusual feature since primates other than man do not readily become infected with the true myxoviruses. Nevertheless, it is the considered opinion of leading students of the influenzas, such as Burnet (1962), Beveridge (1977) and others that new pandemic strains of influenza A viruses arise as zoonoses. The ultimate proof that such occurs in nature is still lacking, but experimental proof supports it as do surveys of the incidence of Influenza A and the distribution of surface antigens in nature.

The Antigenic Structure of Myxovirus A in Different Species

Table 5 shows the antigenic types of Influenza A viruses in man since 1889. The type of influenza in the 1889 pandemic was determined by testing stored sera taken from elderly people in the 1950s. By this means the H antigen was determined to be H3, as in Hongkong Flu, but the N antigen could not be decided.

Table 5 reveals various anomalies. The most important of these is the reappearance in the 1968 Hongkong virus of a different H antigen, but the same N antigen as Asian 1957. In spite of sharing one antigen with the previous pandemic strain, Hongkong virus spread in pandemic fashion though its effects were less severe than usual. The H3 antigen

TABLE 5

Antigenic types of Influenza A viruses in man since 1889

Myxovirus type	Haemagglutinin	Neuraminidase
Hongkong (?) (1889)	H3	??
Spanish Flu (1918)	H1	N1
London (1933)	H1	N1
Melbourne (1946)	H1	N1
Asian (1957)	H2	N2
Hongkong (1968)	H3	N2

recurred after eighty years. It can hardly have survived all this time without causing some epidemics somewhere and so must have been reintroduced from some source. Meanwhile the virus of Spanish Flu survived to cause epidemics from 1933 to 1946, in addition to smouldering in Shopes' pigs.

The survival of the same sub-type of myxovirus between pandemics is assisted by the great antigenic lability of these viruses, which occurs not only in the natural host between epidemics but can be readily induced in virus grown in eggs or tissue culture if exposed to antibody. The results are relatively minor changes of antigenic structure, due to variations of amino acid sequences. Such changes are termed "antigenic drift"; in consequence the same sub-type can reinfect persons, such as the elderly, in whom immunity is weak. Such changes are of a different order from those found in a new pandemic sub-type, in which the surface antigens are completely changed and to which former influenza patients have no immunity whatever. This is known as "antigenic shift". There are three theories as to how this could happen: —

1. *The Mutation Theory.* No competent virologist today believes that an antigenic change of this magnitude in two antigens could occur simultaneously, and the theory need not be further discussed here.

2. *The Adaptation Theory.* This theory states that owing to some mutation an animal virus succeeds in jumping the species barrier and acquires the ability to infect man. This theory postulates a

zoonotic origin for new human influenzas and there is some suggestive evidence to support it. For example, a human virus could pass to an animal reservoir such as a horse or a pig (*vide* Shope's pigs) and re-emerge in man.

3. *The Hybridization Theory*. This theory supposes that an influenza patient becomes transitorily infected also with an animal myxovirus A and that, in the course of replication within the cell, gene exchange occurs between the two viruses so that new viruses with new surface antigens and changed host specifities appear. That this can happen has been proved both *in vivo* and in tissue culture and the theory is supported by surveys of the distribution of H and N antigens in animal hosts. Table 6, showing such distributions as determined to date, is taken from Beveridge (1977).

Twenty three sub-types of myxovirus have been discovered so far, three from man, two from horses and eighteen from birds. The antigens from human and equine sub types have *all* been found in birds. H1 has been found in chickens in Scotland and in terns in South

TABLE 6

Sub-types of Influenza A

Host	First Isolated	H Antigen	N Antigen
man	1933 London	1	1
man	1957 Asia	2	2
man	1968 Hongkong	3	2
swine	1930 Iowa	1	1
horse	1956 Prague	eq1 (av1)	eq1
horse	1963 Miami	eq2 (3)	eq2
chicken	1927 Indonesia	av1 (eq1)	eq1
chicken	1934 Rostock	av1 (eq1)	1
chicken	1949 Germany	av2	eq1
duck	1956 England	av3	av1
duck	1956 Czechoslovakia	av4	av1x
chicken	1959 Scotland	av5 (1)	1
tern	1961 South Africa	av5 (1)	av2
turkey	1963 Canada	av6 (3)	eq2
duck	1963 Ukraine	av7 (3, eq2)	eq2
turkey	1963 England	av1 (eq1)	av3x
turkey	1965 Massachusetts	av6	2
quail	1965 Italy	av2	eq2
duck	1966 Italy	av2	2
duck	1968 Germany	av6	1
turkey	1968 Ontario	av8	av4
shearwater	1971 Queensland	av6	av5
duck	1973 Germany	2	av2
duck	1974 Tennessee	av3	av6

eq = equine; av = avian; no prefix = human.

Africa; H2 has been found in ducks in Germany; H3 is present in turkeys in Canada and ducks in the Ukraine. Human N1 occurs in chickens in Rostock, in Scotland and in ducks in Germany; N2 has been found in turkeys in Massachusetts and ducks in Italy. Human H3 is equivalent also to eqH2. Each sub-type is composed of different combinations of ten H antigens and ten N antigens so far discovered.

In horses, influenza appears to be a rather recent disease. There was a global pandemic in 1956, caused by a virus strain first typed in Czecho-Slovakia, named "Prague Virus". The antigenic structure was defined as H eq1 N eq1; H eq1 is equivalent to H av1. A further pandemic first appeared in Florida in 1963, the viral sub-type being called "Miami Virus". This had the constitution H eq2, N eq2, both antigens being different from those of the Prague virus. In this case, H eq2 = H3, that is Hongkong of man = H av7. The neuraminidase equivalents are:— for Prague N av2, which has been isolated from turkeys; the N antigen from Miami virus has been recovered from chickens and ducks. In 1974, a respiratory disease of horses was reported from Mongolia, in which three Influenza A viruses were implicated:— (i) H av3, N av1; (ii) H av4, N av1; (iii) H av1, N av1. How this strange situation arose is still a mystery.

In pigs, apart from the Iowa infection with Spanish Flu H1, N1, Hongkong influenza, H3 N2, appears to have spread widely in China, Czecho-Slovakia and elsewhere. There is some evidence also that H3 N2 influenza has also infected cattle. Lvov, quoted by Beveridge (1977) isolated the virus from a sick calf in USSR, and cow sera from Uzbekhistan contained low titres of antibody against the virus in 5% to 10% of sera tested. In other parts of the world, no positive results have been obtained from cattle. Lvov also found some fur-seal sera positive for both A and B viruses.

The experimental infection of Bonnet Macaques (*Macaca radiata*), followed by natural spread, has been mentioned above. A more disturbing report of non-human primate involvement came in 1974 from the Southwest Foundation for Research and Education in San Antonio, Texas. During the course of routine virus isolations H3 N2 Hongkong virus was isolated from a group of twenty baboons (*Papio cynocephalus*). None of the baboons was clinically infected. Some baboons were positive on arrival; others became positive later. The original infection must, therefore, have been acquired before shipment and at the time of arrival it must have been passing actively from animal to animal.

In birds, influenza viruses have been recovered from a great many species. Amongst domestic birds, chickens, ducks and turkeys can harbour virus. Amongst wild birds, water birds have been most extensively studied and recoveries have been made from, amongst others, teal, mallard, geese, coot, gulls, tern, shearwater, herons and cormorants. Amongst other wild birds, passerines and psittacines, pigeons and others have yielded virus. It is probably true to say that all birds can, or do, harbour myxoviruses or suffer from infection at some time. Since there are some 8500 avian species and the world population of birds may be 100 000 million, a considerable reservoir of Influenza A viruses must be supposed to exist and the potential for new antigenic hybrids is considerable.

Isolations of virus have been mostly made from healthy birds, which have been trapped, and it is evident that they are chronic carriers of virus, as with Shope's pigs, rather than suffering from active infection. Virus, too, is more readily isolated by swabs taken from the cloaca than from the throat, indicating that the main target organs of the virus may be other than the respiratory tissues. The evidence suggests that many species of birds may be chronic shedders of myxoviruses throughout their lives and that virus will be present in the droppings and could contaminate food or pasture. Birds are the common denominator for all antigenic sub-types of myxovirus A and, in the absence of evidence to the contrary, must be regarded as the origin of new pandemic sub-types of virus. New pandemics mostly originate in isolated areas of the Far East in USSR or China, where relationships of man with wildlife are intimate; this circumstance would favour the hybridisation theory as against the adaptation theory.

The Significance of Pandemic Diseases

Plague pandemics have served during historical times to adjust human population numbers to resources, Influenza pandemics have at times taken a frightening toll of life and could well do so again. It is said that, under modern conditions, a new pandemic of plague could not occur. This view could be over-optimistic; immunity is short-lived and the organism could easily become resistant to drugs and antibiotics. Loss of life during influenza pandemics has not so far approached that caused by plague, yet Fowl Plague caused by a myxovirus kills nearly 100% of chickens, and none can tell whether some new influenza sub-type might not do the same to man. Man is again in a situation of increasing numbers and diminishing resources; he could well prove powerless to prevent adjustment by some pandemic disease.

CHAPTER 4

Infectious Causes of Cancer

Introduction

In the first part of this book, we have traced a new disease pattern in the human race which has evolved since man began to live in crowded communities. We have traced the evolution of new infectious diseases, peculiar to man though derived from animal predecessors. We shall see how in some instances, such as typhus, the purely human disease exists alongside an intermediate stage which can still infect both man and the animals from which it was derived.

It is relevant now to enquire whether there exists today any major area of human disease, which evidence suggests may prove to have: — (i) an infectious origin, and (ii) if so, may have been derived from animals in the past or is likely to be caused by cross-infection from animals today? In modern western societies, the majority of deaths are associated with cardiovascular disease. There has never been any suggestion that such diseases have any form of infectious cause. Second to cardiovascular disease comes cancer, some forms of which, such as the leukaemias and breast cancer, are on the increase to such an extent as to cause profound anxiety. It has been proved that all comparable cancers, which have so far been studied in animals from birds and mice to lower primates, are caused in one way or another by viral pathogens and there is strong circumstantial evidence that the same is true of man. Much of the evidence is so recently acquired and the epidemiology of viral cancers so complex, that the situation is little known or comprehended. A very brief survey is given here in the belief that within a few years some of the cancers will emerge as amongst the most important infectious diseases and that transfer of these diseases from animals will prove important also.

Literature

The literature on viral cancer is so vast as to render worthless any attempt at comprehensive documentation. Two books are of especial value: — "Oncogenic Viruses", by Ludwik Gross, 2nd edition (1970), and "Viruses, Evolution and Cancer", by (eds) Edouard Kurstan and Karl Maramorosch (1974). The subject is also reviewed annually in the US "The Virus Cancer Program', of which I have used the 1975, 1976 and 1977 volumes.

Oncogenic Viruses

The Mechanisms of Malignancy

In their relationships with cells they enter, viruses exist in one of three states: — (i) *Replication* is the normal state; complete new viral particles are manufactured and shed and the cell is destroyed. (ii) *Latency.* When a virus is latent in a cell, replication is inhibited, and the virus survives in the cell without its external coat or "capsid". The genome enters the nucleus and displaces a segment of host DNA. The viral genome becomes integrated with the host genetic material and is reproduced, when the cell divides, as if it were host DNA. If present in the reproductive cells, the viral DNA is passed by either parent to the embryo. Replication of complete new virions is inhibited, but under certain conditions, can be reactivated. (iii) *Transformation.* A transformed cell is a malignant cell. Replication of complete virions is inhibited, but there is interference with the normal activities of the host cell, which multiplies in an uninhibited fashion. In the latent stage, the virus, under special circumstances, may revert to the replicatory stage or to the transforming.

Transformation is genetically determined by viral genes. However, not all viruses, even those of a single group, possess the information to cause transformation; furthermore, it has been shown that information for transformation and replication is situated on different viral genes. It is further known that, when viral genomes become integrated in a host cell, some genes may be shed and the virus may reside in an incomplete form, lacking the power to replicate or lacking the power to transform. For example, the Oncorna C viruses, which cause diseases of the Fowl Leukosis complex, are complete and infection in a susceptible breed of fowl results in malignant disease. The related viruses, which cause the fowl sarcomas, are incomplete and will not cause sarcomas unless one of the leukaemia complex viruses is also present. In this case, the sarcoma virus acquires the lacking information from the leukaemia virus; development of leukaemia is prevented and sarcomas appear.

The implications are important. An inactive virus integrated with the host genome can readily acquire information from a superinfecting virus enabling it either to replicate or transform. Alternatively, a superinfecting virus can acquire transforming information from viral genes in the host genome. Some of the mysteries and difficulties attendant on the study of viral cancers have resulted from this complex situation, and reports from the US (1976 and 1977) "Virus Cancer Program" stress that the search is no longer for oncogenic viruses, but for viral information in host DNA.

Cancer of viral origin may, then, develop in the following circumstances: — (i) if a latent virus is activated by a co-carcinogen, radiation or chemical; (ii) if a new virus acquires transforming information from viral genes already present; (iii) if an incomplete resident virus acquires transforming information from a new virus. Such new viruses could be acquired either from human or animal sources. Viral cancers can, therefore, be justly regarded as potential zoonoses. However, of the four viral groups concerned with the causation of cancer in animals, only one, that of the oncornaviruses, appears likely to be implicated in this way.

The Groups of Viruses Responsible for Causing Cancer

The four groups of viruses responsible for causing cancer are: — 1. The Papova group; 2. The Adenovirus group; 3. The Herpes group; 4. The Oncornavirus group.

The Papova Group. This group consists of the papilloma viruses, mouse parotid tumour virus (polyoma) and simian SV40. In the early stages of infection, the tumours caused appear to be non-malignant in that they cannot be transplanted and do not metastasize. Tumours are benign and self-limiting in size or may regress. Sometimes, they become malignant, possibly because of superinfection with a virus of some other group. They are very small viruses with a core of single-stranded DNA. There is no evidence that any human tumour is caused by any papovavirus of animal origin, though genetic information related to SV40 has been detected in several human tumours.

The Adenovirus Group. The adenoviruses are similar to papova, but slightly larger. Three strains of human adenovirus, numbers 12, 18 and 31 contain transforming information and are strongly oncogenic in rodents, as are 5 of 17 simian strains. They do not, however, appear to be oncogenic in man and there is no evidence that any human tumours are derived from adenoviruses acquired from animal sources. Adenoviruses can hybridize with SV40 and such hybrids have been given inadvertently to a million human beings in adenovirus vaccines. No cases of neoplasia resulted.

The Herpesviruses. Two herpesviruses, *H. saimiri* and *H. ateles*, which are natural pathogens of squirrel and spider monkeys respectively, cause rapidly progressive fatal leukaemias, lymphomas and sarcomas in closely related monkey species. Man is susceptible to infection with *H. simiae*, a natural pathogen of macaque monkeys, which causes an almost invariably fatal ascending myelo-encephalitis. However, there is no evidence that any herpesvirus acquired from an animal source is oncogenic in man. There is strong evidence that man's own latent herpesviruses are associated with some common neoplastic conditions. *H. simplex* type 2 is widely associated with cervical carcinoma of women and has been suggested as a cause of carcinoma of the prostate in men; it is venereally transmitted, being present in semen. Another herpesvirus, the Epstein Barr Virus (EBV) causes Infectious Mononucleosis or Glandular Fever. The target organs of the virus are the B lymphocytes, which are transformed in the patient and remain transformed throughout life, even when active symptoms have subsided. The disease is, therefore, a low grade, self-limiting, leukaemia of the B lymphocytes, the only neoplastic disease of man so far fully proven to be of infectious origin. EBV is also constantly associated with the well known Burkitt Lymphoma of African children and with naso-pharyngeal carcinoma of eastern Asia; there is little doubt that it is the cause of both. All herpesviruses, whether oncogenic or not, have properties of latency. They are large viruses, in which the core contains double-stranded DNA.

The Oncornaviruses. The oncornaviruses all possess transforming ability. In birds, there are five sub-types, A, B, C, D and E, distinguished by the particle morphology and other properties. Only B and C are of importance in mammals and so potentially in man. These viruses contain RNA and multiply by budding when attached to the host cell plasma membrane. Their oncogenic properties are thought to be due to induced chemical and morphological changes in this membrane, so that cell multiplication ceases to be regulated by "contact inhibition". The viruses also possess a gene for the manufacture of an enzyme — a polymerase — known as "reverse transcriptase", by which DNA copies of themselves are constructed. In the DNA or "provirus" form, viral genes become integrated in the host DNA, as described above. Intact viral genomes or viral genetic information can be demonstrated in virtually all mammalian cells including human.

Type B oncornaviruses are the cause of breast tumours of mice; they are frequently present in human milk and can be found in a great many cases of breast tumour tissue in women. There seems little doubt that they are the cause of breast cancer in women the development of which is also hormone dependent. Type C oncornaviruses are the cause of leukaemias, lymphomas and sarcomas in birds, rodents, cats, dogs, cattle, horses and other animals including simian primates. Type C particles are widely associated with similar neoplasms in man.

Oncornaviruses are transmitted in three ways: — (i) vertically in the sex cells; (ii) horizontally shortly after birth as with mammary carcinoma of mice transmitted by the milk; (iii) horizontally at a later stage *post-partum*. When the viruses are transmitted horizontally, antibodies against them can be readily detected. With vertically transmitted virus, antibody is weakly developed, because the foetus has acquired tolerance during development.

The antigenic relationships of the oncornaviruses of different mammalian species suggest that oncornavirus DNA has been handed down vertically generation to generation for at least 40 million years, evolving *pari passu* with the host. These relationships reflect also the taxonomic relationships of the host species. They may also suggest that certain oncornaviruses may originally have been acquired from other species by horizontal transmission. For example, Harvey Rabin (1978) states that non-human primate oncornaviruses closely resemble those of a wild-living Asiatic mouse, but are far removed from those of the house mouse; he suggests their derivation from those of the Asiatic mouse.

The malignant and, where complete, replicatory properties of latent oncornaviruses can be potentiated by ionizing radiation and by oncogenic chemicals; studies with mouse tissues show that, even when malignancy is induced by these means, viruses with transforming ability appear in them; this proves that the role of the carcinogenic agent is that of a co-carcinogen and not a primary one.

The subject will not be further pursued here. Enough has been said to show that there is strong evidence: — (i) that many human neoplasms are the result of the presence of viruses or viral genetic information; (ii) that in some cases exogenous viruses are responsible; (iii) that such exogenous viruses may be derived from animal sources, in some cases serving to recombine with endogenous human viruses. These suggestions may appear speculative, but it is difficult to believe that alone in the animal kingdom human neoplasms are not associated with infectious causes.

PART II
The Major Zoonoses of Modern Society

CHAPTER 5

The Arboviruses

The Natural History of Arboviruses

The arboviruses are a group of infectious agents that are transmitted by arthropod vectors, in which they have the ability to multiply. Some 230 have been identified and more continue to be discovered. A number, possibly most, infect birds from which they come to infect other vertebrates — mammals and even rattlesnakes — by way of the bite of an intermediate host. A number come to infect man in this way, some being of great importance. Infection is often inapparent in an accustomed host, though antibody production is provoked. In other hosts, a febrile disease is caused which, if not fatal, leaves a durable immunity. This does not necessarily mean that arbovirus diseases are density dependent, because the viruses can live and multiply in the arthropod vector and many can pass to the next generation by transovarian infection. In some cases the arthropod is more than a vector, forming the reservoir of infection which enables the virus to survive. Most arboviruses have two components, one viscerotropic and the other neurotropic. Due to the latter, nervous involvement is a feature of many of the diseases leading to various forms of paresis and paraplegia, from which recovery may be only partial. The chief vectors are mosquitos or ticks, though sometimes sandflies (Phlebotomus spp.) are involved and bird mites are known to harbour virus; the latter are not believed to play an important part in non-avian hosts. For reviews, see Andrewes (1964), Burnet (1962), and in primates, Fiennes (1967) and Felsenfeld (1972).

The arboviruses have been placed in three major groups A, B and C. Group B viruses are responsible for the most important diseases that affect man; all are zoonoses. Most important of all is Yellow Fever, which has played an important role in human history. The natural history of yellow fever was established after decades of devoted work in Africa and South America by teams of scientists working under the auspices of the Rockefeller Institute in New York. In the course of screening animals for evidence of yellow fever infection, a number of hitherto unknown viruses of both A and B groups were identified, some of importance in human medicine. Because of their importance, we shall consider the B group viruses first with special reference to Yellow Fever, Dengue and the Russian Spring-Summer Complex.

The Natural History of B Group Arboviruses

Nobody knows how many B arboviruses there may be which are occasionally passed to human hosts from animals. The accidental discovery of a number during routine yellow fever screening suggests that there may be a great many. In illustration of the point, two such will be mentioned here, one from Africa and one from South America: — West Nile Virus and Ilhéus Virus.

West Nile Virus. The West Nile Virus was first isolated at the Yellow Fever Institute at Entebbe, Uganda. It was subsequently found to be widespread and important, having a distribution in Egypt, Uganda, South Africa, probably other parts of Africa, Israel and India. In Egypt, it is endemic, usually causing a silent infection in children. In other parts, especially Israel, it causes a short febrile illness, with headache, glandular swellings, maculo-papular rash, sore throat and limb pains. The natural hosts are probably birds, but antibodies to the virus have been found in different parts of Africa in sera of human beings, monkeys, domestic animals and birds. It is transmitted by culicine mosquitos, but bird ticks too have been found to carry and transmit infection.

Ilhéus Virus. The Ilheus Virus, too, was discovered during routine screening for yellow fever, but in South America not Africa. It has a distribution in Brazil, Colombia, Central America and the Caribbean. In man, it causes infection which is usually inapparent, but sometimes encephalitis develops. The natural hosts are birds, though some mammalian species, including horses, become infected. It is transmitted by several species of mosquitos.

Yellow Fever — Historical

The history of yellow fever has been reviewed by Burnet (1960, 1962) and by Fiennes (1964). The disease in man occurs in two different forms — jungle and urban. Jungle yellow fever is the parent form, of which a great deal is now known but it is the urban form, which has been important historically. This form of infection is transmitted in human populations by man to man infection through the intermediate host, the common urban mosquito, *Aedes aegypti*, which enjoys an almost worldwide distribution. The incubation period in man is from three to six days and the infection may be mild, severe or fulminating. In severe outbreaks the mortality may be as high as 40%. There are two stages to the disease. The onset of the first stage is sudden, and it is accompanied by high fever, nausea, vomiting and constipation, with aches and pains in stomach and limbs. At the end of this stage, the temperature falls and the second stage begins, marked by a tendency to haemorrhages. The liver becomes involved and there is severe jaundice accompanied by urinary retention; black coloured blood is vomited. Severe prostration occurs as the symptoms become intensified. Death occurs in 4-10 days after onset.

Such was the disease which, in West Africa and the New World became the most feared of all. It was formerly endemic in West Africa, being continually reintroduced from jungle sources. This disease, more than any other, earned for West Africa the reputation of being the white man's grave and prevented white settlement there: —

"Beware, my son, the Bight of Benin,
Whence few come out, though many go in."

From West Africa the disease was transported to the New World by mosquitos harbouring in the slave ships; as a result both jungle and urban types became established. Outbreaks associated with ships have appeared in many parts of the world: Gibraltar, 1818; St. Nazaire in France, 1861; Swansea in Britain, 1865; Memphis, 1878; New Orleans, 1905. A description of yellow fever, as it occurred at the siege of Cartagena in 1740 is to be found in "Roderick Random" by Tobias Smollet. Other outbreaks have occurred in Brest, Rochfort, Portland Maine, Halifax (Nova Scotia) and Boston (Massachusetts). The epidemics were all associated with sea ports; the disease, however, in no case became permanently established and is evidently not self-perpetuating unless refreshed from a jungle source.

Existence of yellow fever in the island of Haiti led to one of the most momentous events in history. Because of the mortality amongst their troops, the French abandoned the island in face of an uprising of negro slaves led by a remarkable former coachman, Toussaint l'Ouverture. Without a base in Haiti, the French were unable to maintain communications with their North American colony of Louisiana and the port of New Orleans. Consequently, the emperor Napoleon Bonaparte, in 1803, sold Louisiana to the United States in the biggest real estate deal of all time, known as the Louisiana Purchase. As well as the present State of Louisiana, the French colony at the time comprised the entire Mississippi and Missouri valleys as far north as Oregon. This deal achieved the emperor's purpose of denying New Orleans to the British, who otherwise would undoubtedly have seized it. Had they done so, the Anglo/American war of 1812 would never have taken place.

The Natural History of Yellow Fever

Documented reviews of yellow fever are given by Fiennes (1967) and by Felsenfeld (1972). Jungle Yellow Fever had its origins in Africa and is caused by a commensal virus of mosquitos inhabiting the upper canopy of the evergreen forests of central tropical Africa. Virus has on occasions been isolated from male mosquitos, which do not take blood meals, indicating that passage through a mammalian host is not necessary for its perpetuation. In Africa, the virus is specific to mosquitos of the genus *Aedes* and the common carrier is *A. africanus.* Monkeys inhabiting the upper forest arcades become infected by mosquitos at an early age; they pass through a mild disease, virtually symptomless and develop immunity. Viraemia rarely persists for more than six days, and it is during this period that the new generation of mosquitos becomes infected. The virus can never be isolated from recovered monkeys, although antibodies can be demonstrated in the blood serum. Therefore, the mosquito, not the monkey, forms the reservoir of the virus, a situation which could well be true of other arboviruses also. The human disease is acquired from another mosquito, *A. simpsoni*, which migrates diurnally from the treetops to ground level and feeds on both monkeys and man. Persons infected in this way introduce infection to the urban mosquitos, *A. aegypti* and an urban cycle of the disease, with man to man infection, is started.

In the forests of South and Central America, yellow fever virus became established in two genera of mosquitos, *Sabethes* spp. and *Haemagogus* spp., in which it was able to form a reservoir. Both genera feed normally on monkeys at treetop level, but may occasionally descend to the ground. However, the lumber industry is of importance in these parts and, when a tree is felled, the mosquitos are brought down in clouds and viciously attack the lumberjacks, who acquire the jungle infection and start an urban epidemic. Unlike the African monkeys, some of the New World species succumb to yellow fever and mortality may be high. The disease occurs in epidemics, which frequently coincide with epidemics in man.

The Natural History of Dengue

The dengue virus is closely related to that of yellow fever, and some virologists believe that it was evolved from it. It is surprising, in view of the ease with which yellow fever became established in the New World, that it never appeared in eastern countries. However, the virus exists in two sub-types 1 and 2 and shows the property of "antigenic drift" (as with influenza) which suggests that yellow fever may have appeared in eastern countries and the dengue virus evolved from it. In general, dengue occurs in places from which yellow fever is absent, such as the Middle East and Mediterranean, Japan, Australia, New Guinea, Fiji and Formosa. It occurs in epidemics, which resemble those of influenza in speed of development and morbidity rate. Epidemics recur at intervals, because immunity to the disease is somewhat weak. Table 7, from Burnet (1962), shows the frequency of epidemics from 1889 to 1943.

TABLE 7
Distribution of Dengue during periods of major prevalence

1889-90	Middle East and Mediterranean. Egypt and East Africa
1906-07	Texas, Cuba, Soudan, Phillipines, Australia, Fiji
1916	Bermuda, Middle East, Formosa, Australia
1922	Southern states of USA, Japan
1926-28	Greece and Middle East, Aden, Australia, New Caledonia
1942-43	Australia, Hawaii, New Guinea

The disease is transmitted by mosquitos and appears to maintain itself endemically in human populations by direct man ——→ mosquito ——→ man transmission. Wildlife hosts are also suspected for it, such as monkeys and other arboreal animals in Malaya and flying foxes and fruit bats in Australia. It is believed that a wildlife reservoir must play a part in its epidemiology, but this is still not established. Its serological position, also, is still too uncertain for its relationship to yellow fever to be certainly established.

The Russian Spring-Summer Complex of Tick-borne Arboviruses

This group of diseases is well reviewed by van der Hoeden (1964). Amongst the group B arboviruses is a number, which are tick-borne and have some interest as zoonoses. They are grouped together, being rather similar, as the "Russian Spring-Summer Complex". Among them are:— (i) Russian Spring-Summer Encephalitis; (ii) Central European or Biphasic Meningo-Encephalitis; (iii) Louping Ill of sheep; and (iv) Kyasanur Forest Disease. Diseases of this group are all transmitted by ticks of the family Ixodidae and are antigenically closely related. They differ, however, in their pathogenicity to man, pathology, vectors and cycles in nature.

Russian Spring-Summer Encephalitis. The wildlife reservoir of Russian Spring-Summer Encephalitis is to be found in wild rodents and possibly also in birds. The vector is the tick *Ixodes persulcatus* and infection is passed to human patients, mostly adult males, by their bites. The disease appears in April and reaches an epidemic peak in late May or early June; it disappears again at the end of June. The main victims are persons working in virgin forests, such as foresters, lumbermen, hunters and road builders. The disease is occasionally mild or inapparent, but more often the consequences are severe with a death rate of 5% to 30% from encephalitis. After an incubation period of 8-18 days, there occur fever, headache, nausea, vomiting and pains in the neck. Symptoms of meningitis appear next with rigidity of the neck and often paralysis of the muscles of the limbs, neck and back; in fatal cases the muscles of respiration may be involved. Death occurs in 4-7 days from onset. Recovered patients may be permanently afflicted by partial paralyses. The disease occurs in forested areas of north Russia and Siberia.

Central European or Biphasic Meningo-Encephalitis. This disease commonly occurs in many central European countries, Czecho-Slovakia, Germany, Yugoslavia, Austria, Hungary, Poland and Bulgaria; it has also been reported from Sweden, Finland and European USSR. The disease is contracted from tick bites, chiefly *Ixodes ricinus*, but can also be acquired from drinking the milk of infected goats. The viral reservoir is to be found in wild rodents, from which either goats or man can be infected if bitten by a tick carrying the virus. The human disease is said, in Yugoslavia, to be caused mainly by tick bites; in other countries, especially the USSR, infection is mostly acquired from goats' milk. The disease occurs most commonly in young or middle-aged persons from peasant families living in woodland areas. Widespread epidemics often occur, in which the disease tends to be mild with few reported deaths and only rarely permanent residual nerve impairment. The course of the disease is somewhat characteristic. Influenza-like symptoms, with mild meningeal involvement, occur after 4-21 days from infection by tick bite or consumption of infected milk. There are headache, vomiting, anorexia, abdominal pains and stiff neck. After 3-5 days, the temperature returns to normal and the disease becomes quiescent for 4-20 days. The second stage, a meningo-encephalitis, then suddenly appears with high temperature, severe headache and frequent or incessant vomiting. Mild cases show somnolence and mental confusion; the more severe, coma and delirium; symptoms of encephalitis and encephalo-myelitis develop with various areas of paralysis.

Louping Ill. Louping Ill is primarily a disease of sheep, which occurs in epidemics in Scotland, northern England and Ireland. It is of economic importance, because of the numbers of sheep lost. Naturally acquired infections in man are rather rare, though laboratory workers are at risk because infection can be acquired through the respiratory system. The course in sheep is biphasic as with the Central European disease; a febrile disease is followed after an interval by involvement of the central nervous system with an acute encephalo-myelitis. In man, the disease also runs a biphasic course but is usually mild, though recovery is slow. Sheep appear to constitute the sole reservoir of the virus, since no wild animal has so far been implicated. It is transmitted by the nymphal stage of *Ixodes ricinus*.

Kyasanur Forest Disease. Documented accounts of Kyasanur Forest Disease are given by Fiennes (1967) and by Felsenfeld (1972). The disease was first identified in late 1955 in the Kyasanur Forest area of the State of Mysore in south western India. A large number of Bonnet Macaque Monkeys (*Macaca radiata*) and langurs (*Presbytis entellus*) were found dead in the forest. During the next year, there occurred a severe prolonged febrile disease in a number of people living in the area; this was called the "monkey disease" by the natives. The outbreak lasted three months, and a second outbreak began early in 1957 over a wider area. The virus was identified as belonging to the Russian Spring-Summer Complex, and the transmitting agent was found to be a tick, *Haemaphysalis spinigera*. Haemaphysalis are three host ticks; at each moult, larva to nymph, nymph to adult, the tick falls to the ground and acquires a new host. Larval and nymphal ticks are parasitic on arboreal species, such as monkeys; the adults attack ground-living animals, such as rodents and ungulates. In the monkeys, the disease has a seasonal incidence, being present in the dry weather when the ticks are in the larval and nymphal stages. During the wet season very few ticks are found on the monkeys, but cattle become heavily infested with adult males and females. The cattle are thought to be the source of human infections, but the actual reservoir of the virus is in small wild animals, especially rodents. In man, the disease is biphasic, but both episodes are febrile and involvement of the central nervous system has not been reported. There is a death rate of approximately 10% amongst infected persons resulting from internal haemorrhages and shock.

The Natural History of A Group Arboviruses

The most important of the A group arboviruses are the three equine encephalitides, of which some account will be given. Semliki Forest Virus was isolated in Uganda during the course of yellow fever research, and would be otherwise unknown. It causes symptomless infections in man and antibodies have been found in six species of wild primates in Uganda; it can be transmitted by both anopheline and culicine mosquitos; the reservoir host is unknown. Two similar A arboviruses, which cause unpleasant but not fatal disease in man in Africa, are those of Chikungunya and O'Nyong-Nyong. Both are transmitted by mosquitos, but no hosts other than man have been discovered. Sindbis Virus causes fever in human patients and is widespread, occurring in Egypt, South Africa, India, Malaya, the Phillipines and Australia. The natural hosts are believed to be birds and it is transmitted by culicine mosquitos.

The equine encephalitides are important zoonoses; they are: — Western Equine Encephalitis, Eastern Equine Encephalitis and Venezuelan Equine Encephalitis. All three are transmitted by mosquitos; the natural reservoirs are believed to be birds; the predominant symptoms in all three are associated with the nervous system. There is evidence also that these diseases can be transmitted from horse to horse, presumably also from horse to man, by droplet infection.

Western Equine Encephalitis (W.E.E.)

W.E.E. constitutes a major threat to horses in western states of the USA, and there have been a great many epidemics. During these epidemics, and even between them, epidemics have also occurred in the human populations. One such in the western states of the USA and Canada affected thousands of people and caused a large number of deaths. The disease is transmitted by a predominantly avian mosquito, *Culex tarsalis*, and is commonest in rural areas between May and September. Death rates in horses are some 27%, in man 10%. A febrile phase of the disease is quickly followed by invasion of the nervous system. Adverse sequelae are rare following recovery.

Eastern Equine Encephalitis (E.E.E.)

The Eastern form of the disease is endemic on the eastern seaboard of the USA from New England to Mexico. As with W.E.E., epidemics may be widespread and severe, being coincident in horses and humans. Pheasants are often found to suffer from epidemics at the same time. Death rates are extremely high, often reaching 90% in horses; in man, most cases occur in children under ten years old, in whom the mortality is usually 65% to 70%. The reservoir is believed to reside in wild birds, and transmission from bird to bird is effected by the mosquito, *Culiseta melanura*. This mosquito will not, however, attack either horses or man and the transmitting agent in them is believed to be *Aedes spp.*

Venezuelan Equine Encephalitis (V.E.E.)

The Venezuelan disease causes a high fatality rate in horses but is mild in man. Its range is limited to South and Central America, though one epidemic occurred in Trinidad. In man, there are mild influenza-like symptoms and the nervous system is not involved. The transmitting agent is the mosquito, *Mansonia titillans.* As with W.E.E. and E.E.E., the reservoir appears to be birds, though in most wild birds the infection is symptomless.

Group C and Miscellaneous Arboviruses

The C group arboviruses comprise a few serologically distinct viruses isolated in South America from human beings, monkeys, mice and mosquitos. Infected persons have fever, headache and malaise. Antibodies are found in a proportion of people and forest mammals in the Amazon valley. They are likely to be zoonoses, but little is known of them and they are of no great importance.

There also exist a number of arboviruses in different parts of the world, which are serologically distinct from the three main groups. Of these two are important as zoonoses, Colorado Tick Fever and Rift Valley Fever.

Colorado Tick Fever

Four to five days after the bite of an infected tick, fever develops with chills, aches in head and limbs and often vomiting. Encephalitis may occur, especially in children. Virus has been recovered from several species of wild rodent, mostly from ground squirrels. Infection is transmitted by the tick, *Dermacentor andersoni.*

Rift Valley Fever

Rift Valley Fever is a disease of sheep, goats and cattle, which occurs only in Africa — Kenya, Uganda and South Africa. An epidemic in South Africa in 1951 killed some 100 000 lambs. The main lesions are a massive hepatitis, the liver being of a characteristic golden colour. The virus is, however, pantropic and affected lambs show fever, vomiting, mucopurulent nasal discharge and bloody diarrhoea. In man it resembles dengue and is probably biphasic, it is said to be usually mild though sometimes causing retinal damage. Those of us, working with the disease in sheep in East Africa, were not satisfied with its mildness. Handling tissues from sheep that had died of the disease was extremely hazardous since infection can be acquired from diseased tissue and many laboratory workers become infected with a disease which is by no means pleasant. Natural infection is transmitted by mosquitos, in Uganda *Eratmopodites chrysogaster*, in South Africa *Aedes caballus*.

General Observations

There are a great many other arboviruses, to which both animals and man are susceptible. One or more of these may acquire importance at any time. It has been suggested that the arboviruses originated in arthropods and that their transfer to vertebrate hosts was secondary. If this is so, there must be an unlimited number of these viruses which could potentially be transferred to vertebrate hosts with unforeseeable consequences. They are less to be feared than such pathogens as those of plague and influenza, because their spread can be controlled through the intermediate host. It is, however, disturbing that pneumonic forms of some of these viruses have appeared as with Louping Ill and Eastern Equine Encephalitis. Pneumonic spread of a virus such as E.E.E., with its extreme virulence for man, could easily lead to a global tragedy.

In the next chapter, we shall consider another virus of serious consequence, which has shown a limited capacity for pneumonic spread and which causes 100% death rate in man, that of rabies.

CHAPTER 6

Rabies

General

The importance of rabies in global epidemiology does not lie in the number of deaths it causes, which are comparatively trivial. World Health Organisation statistics, *vide* WHO annual "World Survey of Rabies", record an average of 700 deaths annually reported by contributing countries. However, it is certain that the reported deaths are far fewer than those, which actually occur, and a truer figure might be some 15 000 deaths of which 10 000 occur in India. Even if these figures should be underestimated, they are insignificant in relation to world population numbers, even Indian alone. Rabies acquires its importance from certain features of the disease as follows: —

1. The disease is globally distributed, except for certain countries, Britain, Scandinavia, Australia and New Zealand, where it is strictly controlled:

2. Because of its existence in wildlife reservoirs, it is very difficult to eradicate once established and poses a lasting threat to the health of man and his livestock:

3. In endemic areas, it tends to flare up cyclically and to be spread outwards in epidemic form:

4. Once symptoms have developed, the death rate in man and livestock is 100%. Possible exceptions to this rule are discussed under:

5. Any person bitten by a rabid animal must, even when prophylactic treatment is promptly administered, suffer months of uncertainty before he can be certain that he will not develop rabies:

6. In a proportion of subjects, prophylactic treatment can cause severe cerebral symptoms and even death. When the physician considers the risk of rabies developing to be slight, he will be hesitant about prescribing it:

7. Once rabies has developed, death inevitably occurs after some days of the most appalling agony and apprehension:

8. Once rabies has appeared in a district, it is unsafe to keep dogs and cats unless strictly controlled. Dogs can be confined and muzzled, but this is not so easy with cats. The position has been improved since the widespread use of vaccines in dogs and cats, but such vaccines still do not give 100% protection and their use is attended by some risk.

9. In some South American countries, vampire bat transmitted rabies is the biggest single cause of losses amongst cattle. Losses of domestic stock, including cattle and horses, are not inconsiderable in Europe also.

The literature on rabies, as might be expected, is truly vast. All aspects of the disease are well summarised by Johnson (1959), but this review is somewhat outdated. For a more recent semi-popular account, reference may be made to Kaplan's (1977) "Rabies: the Facts."; though excellent in most ways, this work deals inadequately with rabies in monkeys and bats. For simian primates a comprehensive documented review by Fiennes (1972) appears in Part II of "Pathology of Simian Primates". For the situation in bats, reference should be made to Sulkin and Allen's (1974) "Virus Infections in Bats". An excellent account of rabies as a zoonosis is given by Tierkel (1964) in van der Hoeden's "Zoonoses". The pathology of the disease is well covered by Innes and Saunders (1962) in their "Comparative Neuropathology". I should draw attention also to the classical studies of Hurst and Pawan (1932) describing the pathology of bat transmitted rabies in Trinidad. The epidemiology of rabies in India is described by Ahuja (1958).

All warmblooded animals, including birds, can be infected with rabies, though there is great differential suceptibility. In coldblooded animals, the virus is inactive as it is in animals such as bats, when they are in a state of hibernation. As with plague, two forms of the disease are recognised: (i) *the sylvatic*, in which the infection is endemic and self-perpetuating in hosts which can survive and retain the virus in latent form; (ii) *urban* or epidemic, in which "vectors", such as dogs become infected from "reservoir" hosts and spread the disease. The usual sequel of events so far as man is concerned is: — reservoir host (bat or wild carnivore, e.g. mustelid or fox) ⟶ vector, e.g. wolf, dog or cat ⟶ man. However, in North America many human cases occur from direct contact with animals such as skunks or raccoons. In Africa and elsewhere endemic foci of the disease tend to be discontinuous suggesting that the ultimate reservoir of virus exists in animals that are not uniformly distributed.

The Etiology of Rabies

Rabies is caused by a virus, placed in a group of RNA viruses known as Rhabdoviruses. More than sixty rhabdoviruses have been identified in a wide variety of hosts, such as plants (plantain, potato), insects, fish and other animals; one such is the virus of vesicular stomatitis of cattle. The virus of rabies can parasitize most tissue cells, but causes damage only to certain cells of the central nervous system. It is not spread by the blood and viraemia is exceptional. Replication can occur in salivary gland, muscle and nerve cells. The virus is intensely lipotropic and sites of latency are to be found in fatty tissues, such as the brown fat — the hibernation gland — of bats.

Rabies virus is characteristic in its very slow rate of invasion. It enters the myelin sheaths of voluntary nerves, along which it was formerly believed to progress towards the central nervous system. It is today generally accepted that its progress is along the nerve axons rather than the myelin sheaths, since it is here that virions have been located. Symptoms do not, however, develop until the virus has reached the actual neurones. Hence, the further away from the CNS the source of infection, the longer is the incubation period, head wounds being more dangerous than limb wounds. Furthermore, immunisation procedures are in most cases effective in preventing the spread of the virus if given soon enough after an infected bite. Once the CNS is reached, virus spreads to other tissues, especially the salivary glands; indeed, the saliva can become infective before nervous symptoms develop. Transmission occurs by way of infected saliva either as the result of a bite or from licking abraded skin. Infection may, however, also be spread by inhalation of dried faeces and urine of bats, as sometimes occurs in bat caves.

In man incubation periods of less than fifteen days are very rare; over twelve months are exceptional and said to be suspect in any case. Figures given by Ahuja (1958) for observed cases in India are:— *Bites on Head, Neck and Face* 34 days; *Upper Extremities* 46 days; *Lower Extremities* 78 days. The incubation period was less than a month in 33% of cases; 1-3 months in 49%; 3-6 months in 13%; 6-12 months in 3·5%; over 12 months in 0·5%. The disease, therefore, is unlikely to develop after six months, but might do so even after 12 months.

It was believed until recently that the virus of rabies was serologically unique in the rhabdovirus group. It is now known, however, that there exist a number of "rabies-related" viruses, of which six have been described and defined:—

1. Lagos Bat Virus, isolated from the brain of a fruit-eating bat in Nigeria.

2. Nigerian Horse Virus from a horse which died of a rabies-like disease, known as "staggers".

3. Obodhiang Virus isolated from mosquitos, *Mansonia uniformis* in the Sudan.

4. Kotonkan Virus isolated from midges, *Culicoides sp.*, in Nigeria.

5. Mokola Virus, isolated from the viscera of shrews, *Crocidura sp.*, in Ibadan, Nigeria, and from two human patients in the same area.

6. Duvenhage Virus, isolated in South Africa from the brain of a man, who had apparently died of rabies following a bat bite.

The presence of rabies-like viruses has also been reported from Central Europe in small field rodents, such as the Common Vole, *Microtus arvalis*, the Yellow-necked Mouse, *Apodemus flavicollis*, and the Wood Mouse, *A. sylvaticus*.

Epidemiology of Rabies

Rabies appears to have first become of epidemic significance in Europe, including Britain, from A.D. 1500 onwards. Dogs were affected but also such wild animals as foxes, badgers and bears; the most feared were rabid wolves, the bites of which were regarded as involving the greatest risk. A second major epidemic began early in the eighteenth century, involving wildlife and dogs; this reached Britain in 1735. By the mid-eighteenth century rabies had become prevalent also in North America, especially Boston. A third epidemic in Europe coincided with the Napoleonic wars and persisted for twenty years after; it resembled the outbreak of the 1960s in that foxes were largely implicated and the area involved was similar. Rabies was especially serious in Britain from 1870 to 1903, when it was eradicated; even the deer in Richmond Park became infected. However, in Britain wildlife, including foxes, never became seriously involved for reasons that are unknown. Hence, eradication was possible once correct measures were enforced.

The present epidemic on the continent of Europe had its beginnings after the Second World War. Rabid foxes moved from Poland to East Germany in 1948 and had invaded West Germany by 1950. From there, the disease spread northwards into Denmark, but was eliminated by the eradication of foxes and the maintenance of a fox-free zone north of the German border. Provided that the fox population is kept to less than 1 km^{-2} rabies does not maintain itself, being in this sense density dependent in foxes. From Germany, rabies was carried into France in 1968 and has been spreading slowly towards the Channel coast in spite of rigorous control of fox populations.

The Symptoms of Rabies

The symptoms of rabies are uniquely geared to the spread and survival of the virus. However, although these symptoms become developed in man in their most frightening form, man to man infection virtually never occurs even when the patient in his extremity attacks and bites his attendants. Evidently, man is a dead-end host playing no part in the cycle of infection. There is also no record of rabies being transmitted to a human being by any other primate, though they are potentially dangerous. In them, the symptoms developed in no way suggest the nature of the disease, and many imported monkeys must have died of rabies without the nature of the infection being realised. It would appear probable that in primates, man included, the salivary glands do not become heavily infected; no investigations of the point seem to have been made.

Until neurological symptoms develop, rabies can be forestalled, in man by prophylactic measures and in other animals, even rarely in dogs — by the animal's own immune mechanisms. When this happens, the vector animal becomes immune; in the reservoir animal, the virus may become latent and capable of reactivation in conditions of stress. Once neurological symptoms develop, the areas of the CNS involved are so vital that it is doubtful whether any animal could survive infection even resistant species such as skunks and vampire bats, of which it is known that some succumb. Rabies occurs in two forms known as the "Furious" and the "Dumb" or paralytic. In "furious" rabies the virus becomes located in the brain stem, the limbic system and the hypothalamus. The brain stem contains the cardiac, respiratory and vasomotor centres, and the roots of cranial nerves IX, X and XI, consisting of sensory and motor fibres controlling the tongue and throat. The limbic system, consisting of the amygdaloid nuclei, the hippocampus, the reticular formation and the hypothalamus, is involved in temperature control, co-ordination of the autonomic nervous system and, through control of the pituitary gland, of urinary excretion through the kidneys. In "dumb" or paralytic rabies, the virus attacks the medulla and spinal cord only so that symptoms are less alarming and less conducive to viral spread.

In man and dogs the "furious" form of rabies is commonest, except when infection is derived from bats, when "dumb" rabies develops in man. In dumb rabies, the symptoms are less distressing than in furious, though death invariably occurs from respiratory paralysis within 30 days. Dogs suffering from the dumb form of the disease are easily controlled and less dangerous than those suffering from the furious. The symptoms and course of furious rabies, whether in man, dog, cat or other animal are agonising beyond description. The location of the virus within the nervous system promotes maximum aggression, including sexual. Before paralysis sets in, wolves and dogs lope for considerable distances attacking any living thing and tearing at inanimate objects, such as sticks and stones. They attack without fear, but without fixity of purpose so that their victims are usually mauled but not killed. Dogs usually recognise and respond to the voice of their masters, who may be able to control them and are rarely attacked. Cats attack their masters and anybody else indiscriminately, and are especially dangerous because they fly at the face, the most vulnerable part of the body, with claws and teeth. Dogs have a strange fixity of gaze and gait, which once seen is unmistakeable. I have myself seen only one rabid dog, which I myself had infected by administering live rabies vaccine, evidently insufficiently attenuated, three weeks before. The posture and gaze of the dog were such that I found no difficulty in recognizing the disease, which was subsequently confirmed as true rabies by laboratory methods. The dog was quiet with his owners, but a colleague who attempted to take the dog's rectal temperature was savaged and underwent the hazardous anti-rabies immunisation routine. The owners, although they were not bitten, required the same treatment in case they had been infected by licking.

Man, and man alone, suffers the additional refinement of cruelty, that of "hydrophobia". During the course of the disease, partial paralysis of the throat makes it difficult to swallow, and it might be thought that the fear of water arose from the danger of choking. This, however, is not the case and solid food may be taken, whereas the feel of water in the mouth triggers a violent reaction with tonic spasms and opisthotonus as in tetanus. A similar reaction may be caused also by other stimuli, such as the feel of a draught on the body. The patient avoids drinking for some time for fear of the effects, but eventually becomes unbearably thirsty. Attempts to lift the cup to the lips are thwarted by violent rembling of the arm. Desperate efforts are made to snatch a sip of water, until a last minute terror causes the cup to be flung away and the patient dives beneath the bedclothes. During spasms, the drink or saliva may be coughed out in showers over bystanders. Patients may retch or vomit so violently that tears are caused in the gullet near its junction with the stomach. Cries of alarm may be distorted by paralysis or swelling of the vocal cords which alter the voice so that shouts sound more like barks. The face is a mask of terror; the body racked with tremors or spasms. The patient may struggle frantically to free himself and try to escape from the room; rarely he may attack and bite his attendants. Generalized convulsions, like epileptic fits, may follow, or the patient may go into coma. Even more tragic perhaps, the patient experiences intermissions of normal consciousness and lucidity, when he is fully aware of his circumstances.

The Natural History of Rabies

Rabies reveals many unusual features, which are of interest to the study of disease ecology. It is a zoonosis *par excellence* in the sense that, though there is no obvious reason why it should not be directly transmitted from man to man, it never is transmitted in this way; infection never occurs, except from an animal source. Furthermore, the fatality rate in man is 100%, if we except one single case in which recovery took place, probably assisted by vaccine given too late to prevent the onset of the disease. The same cannot be said of any other disease whether of man or animals. Even myxomatosis at its height killed no more than 99·8% of rabbits, so that some survivors were left to re-establish rabbit populations. The fatality rate from rabies in other animals is not so high as in man, though it is not clear whether this is the result of infections being aborted or from recovery after symptoms have developed. Serological tests have shown that even in wild and domestic Canidae, foxes and dogs, some survive, even though such recoveries have not been actually observed. Such animals remain immune to further attack and there are other species, for example skunks and some bats, of which many do not suffer severely from infection with rabies virus and remain virus shedders. It must be supposed, therefore, that there are reservoirs of the disease in nature, from which epidemics can arise continually.

It was at one time feared that mouse populations of Continental Europe were harbouring the virus, but it appears now that they are unimportant. In many parts of the world, the possible role as viral reservoirs of small wild carnivores, such as Mustelidae, does not appear to have been assessed adequately; meanwhile it is generally accepted that the virus is maintained by epidemic cycles in animals, such as wolves and red, grey and arctic foxes. Since the virus is so lethal to these animals, it is doubtful whether the virus could be maintained in them alone; there must be some reservoir from which lateral spread in epidemic form can take place, even if this exists only in small pockets or foci. In northern Russia, wolves are still believed to be the chief source of infection in a wolf ⟶ dog ⟶ man cycle; but wolves are normally only affected by epidemics at times when their numbers have increased beyond the resources of the habitat; at such times rabies and distemper help to control population numbers and then disappear. Where then do the wolf epidemics originate? In northern Canada, Arctic Foxes are blamed, but they too suffer severely from rabies and the suspicion lingers that the viral reservoir must exist in some other animal. In Africa, rabies is widespread but its distribution is regional, suggesting that it resides in some focus of wildlife that is not unduly affected by it. For example, in Uganda, a country well known to the author from twelve years residence there, rabies was always endemic in the remote West Nile District, home of President Idi Amin, but not elsewhere; from time to time, it would appear in other parts of the Protectorate, but never became endemic.

Jubb and Kennedy (1963) state the problem succinctly: — "Bats are the only vectors known in which rabies is not self-limiting by virtue of being consistently fatal. In all other species the period of communicability is brief." They could have included skunks also, but even so they avoid facing the questions they pose. They state that the reservoir hosts vary from region to region, and within regions from time to time, especially when the disease changes from being endemic to epidemic. They list "reservoir vectors" as: — foxes and skunks in the United States; foxes and dogs in northern Canada, foxes in western Europe, wolves in eastern Europe and Iran, jackals in India and northern Africa, mongoose and genets in South Africa. To lump reservoir and vector together begs the question. The vectors are well known and epidemic rabies can be maintained in them for long periods but eventually the cycle dies back. When outbreaks of rabies occur, it is important that serological surveys of wild animals be undertaken; in this way it can be ascertained what animals have been exposed to infection either clinically or abortively. Some such surveys have been made in the USA, one of which is quoted by Tierkel (1964): —

1. *Fox Sera* 12 + of 262 (4·6%).
2. *Raccoon Sera* 11 + of 196 (5·6%).
3. *Opossum Sera* 2 + of 185 (1·8%).
4. *Bobcat Sera* 5 + of 27 (18·5%).
5. *Skunk Sera* 7 + of 48 (14·5%).

No wild rodents were found to be positive. No attempts have been described to ascertain whether animals showing antibody were carriers of latent virus, so that the possible roles of recovered animals as reservoirs remain undetermined. Nevertheless, both bobcats and skunks come under suspicion. Similar surveys made in South Africa tend to incriminate wild Mustelidae and Viverridae. It is significant, however, that it has never been possible to isolate rabies virus from the salivary glands of foxes, unless neurological symptoms were present. While there is evidence that subclinical immunising infections occur in wild animals in nature, there is no evidence that any animals, except bats, harbour latent virus and shed it over long periods.

Rabies in Bats

The situation with regard to rabies in bats is one of some complexity, of which a detailed account is given by Sulkin and Allen (1974); it is also well summarised by Tierkel (1964). Bats are second only to rodents in numbers of genera and species and are the most abundant of all mammalian Orders. They are also more widely distributed throughout the world than any other mammal, except for man. In spite of this, they are unobtrusive and tend to be unnoticed, a characteristic which is enhanced because many species undergo deep hibernation during the winter months in temperate zones. Bats have, moreover, very diverse food habits and preferences. Some are insectivorous, some fruit-eaters, and the vampires are the only group of vertebrates which allegedly subsist on a sole diet of blood (although in zoos and laboratories they do require other additives). In addition, there are carnivorous Chiroptera, which feed on small mammals, fish, amphibia and reptiles; other species use nectar and pollen as foods. Bats hide away in caves, caverns and hollow trees and also infest human habitations which they contaminate with their urine and faeces.

Bats were first investigated as possible vectors of rabies in southern Brazil in the early 1900s. Deaths of cattle and horses from rabies could not be connected with attacks by wild carnivores or dogs, and an airborne host suggested itself. At the same time, there were reports of bats exhibiting abnormal behaviour — attacking and biting cattle in the daylight hours. Strangely, the first bats to be suspected were fruit bats of the genus *Phyllostoma*. It was not until 1934 that vampire bats (*Desmodus sp.*) were found to be the main transmitters of rabies to cattle in Brazil; this error is so extraordinary that one wonders whether the fruit bats did not in fact initiate the transmission cycle to be superseded later by the vampires; it is impossible to see how the two genera could have been confused. Today the problem is of serious magnitude and has proved very difficult to overcome. In 1956 one million cattle were lost in Brazil alone from rabies, constituting by far the greatest cause of losses. There have been no reports of human deaths resulting from contact with cattle or horses, and vampire transmitted rabies has not been a serious problem in man in South America. However, an epidemic of vampire transmitted rabies occurred in Trinidad in 1929 as described by Hurst and Pawan (1932). Between 1929 and 1937, when the disease was eradicated, 89 persons had died; many of the victims were unaware of being bitten by a vampire. The bats make painless incisions, often in a toe protruding from the bedclothes at night, inducing a flow of blood by means of an anticoagulant present in their saliva, then lapping the blood. The wounds are not easy to detect and there may even be no blood left to mark the site. For some reason unknown, vampire transmitted rabies is usually of the dumb type, as has already been stated. Some vampires show neurological symptoms when infected; they then fly wildly during the day as well as the night and will viciously attack people or animals. It is, however, well established that they often carry asymptomatic infections and transmit rabies virus in the saliva over long periods.

Both vampires and other bat species are now known to be widely infected with rabies throughout the North- as well as the South-American continent from Mexico to Canada; infected bats have not so far been found in Alaska. All genera and species, insectivorous, fruit-eating and blood lapping are involved. Bat rabies was not detected in the United States, until the death of a child from rabies occurred in Florida in 1953 following the bite of an insectivorous bat *Dasypterus floridanus*, and a second bat-induced death occurred in Pennsylvania a few months later. Between then and 1967, infected bats had been found in all of the United States except for Alaska and Hawaii. In Canada rabid bats have been found in British Columbia, Ontario and Manitoba. They are also known to exist in India, Yugoslavia, Hungary, Turkey, Germany and Thailand. Surveys in Indonesia, western and southern Africa, and the United Arab Republic have not so far revealed the existence of bat rabies. However, surveys in the Eastern Hemisphere have been much less intensive than in the West. In 1962, Dr. Constantine, Chief of the South-west Rabies Investigation Station in New Mexico reported two deaths from rabies, one in 1956 and the other in 1958, as a result of entering a large limestone cavern in Texas where rabid bats had been identified. Both men denied having been bitten by bats or other mammals, and it was supposed that they had contracted infection as a result of inhaling infected dust in the musty bat-ridden cave. As a consequence, tests were done by placing native carnivores, foxes, coyotes, raccoons, dogs and skunks in the caverns in such conditions as to exclude the possibility of their being bitten either directly by infected bats or by bat parasites. Some of these animals also contracted rabies, from which it was learned that under certain conditions the disease can be contracted by inhalation of infected material. It is believed that this will only happen, when the concentration of infected material is unusually high as in a bat cave; bat urine and faeces may carry virus.

Investigations, summarised by Sulkin and Allen (1974) have shown that rabies virus can be isolated regularly from apparently healthy bats in endemic areas. This virus proves infectious to other bats of various species, when administered subcutaneously, intramuscularly or intra-nasally. Of the bats infected in this way, a number develop the neurological symptoms of rabies; a number remain asymptomatic although virus can be isolated from the tissues. Bats, therefore, do display the kind of tolerance of rabies virus, which could enable them to be reservoir hosts. The site in the body, where virus is found in highest titre is the "brown fat", the so-called hibernation gland; virus can also be isolated from the nervous system, the salivary glands and the kidneys. During hibernation, the virus remains inactive, though able to initiate overt disease when the animal emerges from its winter sleep. Bat to bat transmission of rabies virus could easily occur by aerosol in bat caves, though they are quarrelsome creatures frequently fighting and biting each other so that direct transmission is also probable. Furthermore, rabid bats, even insectivorous or fruit-eating, will attack and bite other bats or animals and can transmit the disease in this way. Bats are, therefore, undoubted reservoirs of rabies virus and could well be the vectors which carry the disease to small carnivores, some of which (e.g. skunks) could themselves be both reservoirs and vectors. There could thus be a disease cycle: — Bat ⟶ Skunk ⟶ Fox ⟶ Dog or Cat ⟶ Man. Either a dog or cat could well molest a seriously sick bat and be bitten; indeed in the United States at least two of the bat-transmitted cases of rabies occurred in persons who had picked up sick bats and been bitten by them.

The significance of "brown fat" in relation to resident viruses is discussed at length by Sulkin and Allen (1974). Because the rabies virus is so intensely lipotropic, the hibernation gland is ideally suited to retention of the virus in a resting stage during the winter months. Since the Brown Fat is mobilised at the end of hibernation, the virus will be dispersed throughout the body when the temperature rises at the end of winter. These authors also discuss the possible role of this gland and of bats in the overwintering of arboviruses in temperate climates. We have seen that Yellow Fever virus is retained in the mosquitos. With other arboviruses, such as the mosquito-borne encephalitides, hibernating mosquitos have not been found to harbour virus. While active virus has been found in migrating birds in winter, a perfect resting place would also be in the brown fat of hibernating bats. In fact, a number of arboviruses have been isolated from this tissue in bats, which may well prove to have a hitherto unsuspected importance in a number of viral disease cycles.

It is strange that the natural history of so important a disease as rabies is so poorly known. It is difficult to see how a virus that is so highly and universally lethal could maintain itself, unless there existed some species which could act as a reservoir. There are vectors and dead-end hosts galore. Since they all, or almost all, are killed by the virus, from where does the disease reappear in epidemic cycles? It is tempting to say that the recent work on bat rabies has solved the problem. Perhaps it has partially done so, but rabies is rampant in places such as Alaska where apparently there are no infected bats nor are there skunks. The eradication of rabies as a disease of global importance is likely to depend on first solving this conundrum. Meanwhile, the disease continues to spread and extend its range to new areas, causing losses of livestock, deaths and dislocations in most parts of the world. Heaven forbid that the virus should develop properties of spreading by aerosol; such could be the ultimate global tragedy. One thought remains in my mind. Amongst the many misconceptions about this disease, it is said to be universally fatal to man. This is untrue; it is universally fatal, *once neurological symptoms have developed*. There are, or have been, many who have not succumbed to rabies, although they must have absorbed heavy doses of virus; indeed, in persons at risk the incidence of clinical disease is significantly higher in young persons than old. As human beings, therefore, as with dogs and foxes, we have defences against this virus, but cannot eliminate it once it has invaded the central nervous system.

There are other neurotropic viruses which are important as zoonoses, such as pseudo-rabies or Aujesky's Disease. These will not be discussed here, since we are selecting those diseases of especial significance to human disease ecology. The next chapter will, therefore, be devoted to the rickettsioses.

CHAPTER 7

The Rickettsioses

Introduction

The rickettsias resemble viruses in being intracellular parasites, though unlike viruses they are complete organisms possessing both DNA and RNA. Rickettsias are widely distributed in nature particularly in arthropods, from which it is thought that they may have originated. With one exception, all rickettsias pathogenic to vertebrate hosts are, or can be, transmitted by arthropod parasites. While, therefore, the rickettsias are distinct from viruses, neither are they bacteria nor protozoa but constitute an independent group of parasitic organisms. They appear in parasitized cells, usually of endothelial origin, as small rods or spheres in the cytoplasm, very occasionally in the nucleus. They cannot be cultured in cell free media, but grow aerobically in suitable media to which living cells have been added. The rickettsias are named after an American scientist, Ricketts, who died of typhus in 1910 while investigating the disease in Mexico City. It was he who showed in 1906 that Rocky Mountain Spotted Fever, another rickettsial zoonosis, was transmitted by the wood tick and that Mexican typhus was transmitted by lice. The history of human typhus was recorded by the American scientist, Hans Zinsser, in his classical book "Rats, Lice and History", which, though written so long ago as 1935, is still a fund of information on the subject and a delight to read.

Typhus

Typhus is caused by *Rickettsia prowazeki*. Like some other diseases we have been considering, typhus is a "new" disease of man and "density dependent". Though the "classical" form affects man alone, its evolutionary stages as a zoonosis are so clear that its animal origins cannot be doubted. Other rickettsioses are also important as zoonoses.

The Origins of Typhus

A major and enduring review of the rickettsioses is that of Zdrovskii and Golinevich (1960), but Zinsser's (1935) work, based on a life's work on typhus, is crammed with information that would be alien to more specialised accounts of the subject. Human typhus takes two forms: the "murine" or "endemic" typhus and "classical" or "epidemic" typhus. The causal organisms, *R. mooseri* and *R. prowazeki*, are indistinguishable from each other except by laboratory tests. There is, however, a difference of fundamental importance. Murine typhus exists in wild-living rats and mice and can be transmitted to man by rat or mouse fleas, and thence from man to man by lice. It is, furthermore, endemic in certain areas and does not normally cause widespread epidemics. Classical typhus infects only man and is transmitted from man to man by body or head lice (*Pediculus humanus corporis* and *P. h. capitis*), but not by pubic lice (*Phthirus pubis*). It is *R. prowazeki*, which has caused the great typhus epidemics of history which, as we shall see, have caused millions of deaths and profoundly affected the course of history. Typhus is a disease of dirt, squalor and poverty, occurring in conditions of overcrowding and poor hygiene. It has acquired various names such as Camp Fever, Prison Fever and Ship Fever, which denote the typical conditions under which it arises. It follows wars, and warring armies have been destroyed by it. Even in recent times following the Russian revolution, there were between 1917 and 1921 more than twenty five million cases in Soviet territories with up to three million deaths.

Classical Typhus

Classical typhus appears to be a very new disease of man, and the louse is evidently a new agent of transmission. This is shown by the effect of rickettsial infection on the louse itself, which becomes acutely sick and never survives more than 14 days. One might suppose from this that the disease would be self-limiting and would disappear when the last louse died. Up to a point this does happen, since typhus disappears once the conditions of stress have passed and normal hygiene is restored. However, as if by magic it reappears as soon as poor conditions again permit the lice to become re-established. Whereas some persons, who have recovered from typhus, become solidly immune to reinfection, others become "carriers" of the rickettsiae, and may under stressful circumstances again suffer from mild symptoms of typhus. The appearance of mild cases of typhus in the eastern seaboard areas of the United States was for a time a mystery, until it was realised that Brill's Disease, as it was called, only appeared in immigrants who had previously suffered from typhus in their native lands in Europe.

The heyday of typhus is said to have been the eighteenth century. In those not too distant days, the possession of lice in the hair or on the body was the rule rather than the exception; indeed the ancients regarded the presence of lice in their beards as a sign of strength! Within living memory in Britain, children in slum areas were more commonly infested with lice than not, and even today infestation is not uncommon amongst the poorer people. Conditions have, therefore, always been present, in which a resurgence of typhus could occur. There can be no reasonable doubt that the purely human form of typhus has evolved in comparatively recent times from the "murine" by an over-adaptation of the rickettsias to the human host and to the louse as its vector. Should this form disappear, there seems no reason why it should not again be evolved from the murine. Sporadic cases of murine typhus have, no doubt, affected human beings from time immemorial; the disease is endemic in many parts of the world from the Far East to the American continent and gives rise to local epidemics. However, Zinsser finds no evidence of epidemics of classical typhus until the fifteenth century, and this may give evidence of the date at which epidemic or pandemic human typhus was evolved from the murine. Zinsser also discusses at length the association of rats with man; this he regards as of somewhat recent origin also, placing the date at which the black rat arrived in Europe as between A.D. 400 and 1100. Since he regards the mouse as a less dangerous vector of murine typhus than the rat, he considers that conditions were not so conducive earlier for conversion of murine to classical typhus. He quotes Hamilton and Hinton as stating that etymologically the first differentiation of rats and mice is found in the writings of Giraldus Cambrensis, 1146 to 1223, and that after this date the two creatures are clearly distinguished. It was not until later that the brown rat displaced the black.

Symptoms of Typhus

As a disease, typhus presents rather characteristic symptoms, from which it can be recognised even from the inadequate descriptions of diseases given in early writings. It is an acute fever with a typical course, though it sometimes behaves atypically. The onset may be very abrupt, or gradual, the initial stages resembling those of influenza. Temperature rises to 103-104°F., with chills, great depression, weakness and pains in the head and limbs. On the fourth or fifth day after onset a skin rash appears; up to this time diagnosis is difficult, but the exanthemata are characteristic. When the rash appears, the temperature tends to rise further. The rash usually starts on the shoulders and trunk, extending to the extremities, the backs of the hands and feet and sometimes even to the palms and soles. As the exanthemata spread, a severe, often unbearable, headache becomes a feature, more pronounced than in other diseases. Delirium and extreme weakness ensue. However, in mild, endemic cases, especially in children, the rash may be so transient as to pass unnoticed. In the absence of an epidemic and without laboratory aids, typhus often remains undiagnosed, being impossible to differentiate from measles, scarlet fever, typhoid, malaria, and other febrile conditions.

The Importance of Typhus in Human History

An outbreak of disease, which from the accounts of it must have been typhus, occurred in a monastery near Salerno in Italy in A.D. 1083, probably a local epidemic of murine typhus which ran its course and died away. There is no further record of any disease which could be identified as typhus, until it appeared in the armies of Ferdinand and Isabella investing the Moors in the city of Granada in 1489. This epidemic was very severe and had apparently been introduced by mercenaries, who had been fighting for the Venetians against the Turks and were returning from Cyprus to join the Spanish armies. When the army was reviewed at the beginning of 1490, the generals found that 20 000 men were missing from the rolls; of these, 3000 had been killed in action and 17 000 had died of disease. The same disease reappeared in Spain in the year 1557, believed to be derived from the Granada outbreak; it ravaged the Spanish population for 13 years until 1570. At this time also, a severe outbreak of the disease occurred in Mexico City, and was believed transported in naval ships and merchantmen. This belief presents certain difficulties, discussed under. However that may be, there is clear evidence that typhus was well established in Spain during the last decade of the fifteenth century and throughout the whole of the sixteenth, though it was not yet widespread throughout Europe. It was recognised as a new disease by those who had to deal with it and there is no doubt that, so far as Europe was concerned, it had not occurred previously.

By 1528, typhus was playing a decisive role in world history. In that year, the armies of Francis I of France, having devastated Italy and sacked Rome, were investing the Imperial Army of Charles V in Naples. The defending armies were at their last gasp and would have had no hope of resistance for more than a few weeks, had not typhus appeared amongst the French troops numbering some 28 000. Within 30 days, more than half the army had died including the commander, Marshall Lautrec. By the time the siege was raised only 4000 men survived and they were all disarmed or murdered by the local peasantry; none returned to France. As a result, Charles V obtained the mastery of Italy and domination of the Pope, Clement VII. For fear of offending his master, Clement refused to grant the divorce of Henry

VIII of England from his wife, Catherine of Braganza. This refusal led directly to the reformation in England and the dissolution of the monasteries.

It is, on the face of it, unlikely that at this time true classical typhus could have been transported to the New World, for the simple reason that infected lice could not have survived long enough in the old sailing ships. It is, therefore, claimed that the Mexican outbreak must have been murine typhus. Nevertheless, it is a curious coincidence that the serious Mexican epidemic should have occurred at the same time as the first appearance of typhus in Spain. It could surely have arrived in a ship, in which the disease appeared some days out from the home port and ran its course during transit; alternatively, infection could have been derived from a case of Brill's Disease. In spite of claims to the contrary, one must believe that typhus was indeed introduced to the American continent at this time. There is, however, clear evidence that murine typhus was present in South America before the arrival of the conquistadors. Both explanations are possible.

Following its sensational debut in Spain and Italy, typhus spread into France and northwards over the whole of Europe. Having succoured Charles V at Naples, it turned against him and killed more than 10 000 men of his army, which was besieging Metz in 1552. Great numbers died in the military prisons earning for it the name of *Morbus Carcerorum*.

We have seen that the Granada epidemic of typhus was introduced by mercenaries from Cyprus; it is believed that the disease was in fact imported from eastern countries, where it may have been rife a hundred years before it became established in Europe. In those days, the meeting point between east and west lay in the Balkans, and particularly in Hungary where the unfortunate Hungarian kings were endeavouring to stem the Turkish advance with meagre assistance from the Austrian emperors. The Hungarian king, Hunyadi, relieved the siege of Belgrade in 1456, decisively defeating Mohamed II; he was powerfully assisted by a pestilence, the nature of which is uncertain. It was in all probability typhus mingled with plague; the two diseases often appeared together, the one reinforcing the ravages of the other. If typhus was indeed involved, then this antedates the Granada episode. This pestilence struck the Hungarians too, and Hunyadi himself died of it. During the ensuing hundred years, the ceaseless warring continued and the troops brought back pestilence and death with them. In 1542, Joachim, Marburg of Brandenburg, was in Hungary to repel the invaders with an army composed mostly of Germans and Italians. Thirty thousand of his soldiers died of a disease, which this time was undoubtedly typhus. Few Turks or Hungarians died, which strongly suggests that both had formerly been exposed to infection and possessed a degree of immunity. The disease became known as the "Hungarian Disease" and Hungary as the "Graveyard of Germans". Twenty six years later in 1568, this episode was repeated on a yet greater scale under the emperor Maximilian II. The emperor sent a large army into Hungary to protect the eastern borders, and the campaign was achieving complete success. However, the army was encamped on the Danube in intensely hot weather suffering severely from commissariat difficulties. Food was short and inadequate and the men suffered severely from scurvy. Dysentery and enteric fevers weakened resistance and typhus struck in ideal conditions for its development. The death rate was appalling and the whole army disintegrated. The emperor was forced to make an unfavourable peace with the Turks. Typhus spread to Vienna and was carried by the survivors to Italy, Bohemia, Germany and through Burgundy northward into Belgium.

Once well established west of the Balkans, typhus spread over the whole of Europe in pandemic fashion. It was accompanied by plague, smallpox, diphtheria, enteric fevers, famine and continuing savage wars. Zinsser quotes the district physician of Regensburg, Lammert, who chronicled the Thirty Years War from 1600 onwards. He wrote of 1602: —

> There was a severe winter, a cold April, a hailstorm in the summer. The wine was scarce and of poor quality. In this year, there was plague in the Palatinate, through Saxony and Prussia. In Danzig, 12 000 people died in one week. There was a smallpox epidemic in Bohemia; another in Silesia. In southern Germany, enteric fevers raged. There was a famine in Russia accompanied by pestilences of plague and typhus, and in Moscow alone 127 000 people are said to have died of pestilence.

Year by year a similar story is told. The continual reference to the wine harvest in these chronicles is of interest, since it was realised that water was unsafe to drink and, when the wine failed, dysentery and typhoid appeared.

When the Thirty Years War was ended, there was some amelioration of suffering, but typhus was established in all parts of the European continent. Moreover, armed struggle continued in many parts. The Turks still had to be contained, the French invaded the Netherlands and there was widespread famine in Italy. So typhus maintained its grip; even in France there were disastrous epidemics in Poitou and Burgundy in 1651 and 1666. In Russia, Austria and Hungary, the struggle against the invaders continued well into the eighteenth century and typhus remained a continual scourge.

Typhus did not reach Britain, until after it was firmly established on the continent of Europe. However, Britain too was indulging in a civil war; at the siege of Reading in 1643 both armies, parliamentary and royalist, were severely affected by typhus. By 1650, the whole island had been converted by the disease into one vast hospital. Typhus flourished to the greatest extent in the gaols, which were scandalously overcrowded and filthy in the extreme. Conditions remained indescribable until reforms in 1770, and typhus became known as "gaol fever". Typhus occasionally escaped from the gaols and ran riot in the surrounding countryside. This was inclined to happen, when prisoners were brought to court for trial and in some well known cases the courts became known as the Black Assizes. Particularly serious incidents occurred at Oxford in 1577 and at the Old Bailey in 1750.

The Oxford incident is worthy of relation. A catholic book-binder, Rowland Jencks, was committed to prison at Oxford accused of speaking evil of the government, profaning God's word, abusing ministers and staying away from church. In a crowded court, he was condemned to have his ears cut off. Shortly before the trial a number of prisoners had died in their chains; soon after the trial typhus appeared amongst those who had attended it. Sir Robert Bell, the Lord Chief Baron; Sir Nicholas Barham, the Sheriff; the Under-sheriff; and all members of the Grand Jury, except two, died of typhus. Total deaths numbered more than five hundred, one hundred of the stricken being members of the University. Jencks himself escaped infection and settled earless in France.

By the beginning of the eighteenth century, typhus was well established endemically throughout Europe, and invasion from the east could no longer be blamed for epidemic episodes. There were wars of Spanish, Polish and Austrian successions in the first half of the century, every one attended by typhus. The epidemics, which started in the armies, spread throughout central Europe. At the siege of Prague alone 30 000 people died, including all the French medical staff. In Ireland, typhus aggravated the effects of the potato famine in 1740. British armies suffered after Dettingen in 1743 and again in the Spanish wars in 1762. During the Seven Years War, the French Revolution and the Napoleonic wars, there were more casualties from typhus than from martial activities. At the end of the eighteenth century and during the early nineteenth, England suffered from severe epidemics, although the country had been relatively free for some time previously. This series of epidemics is believed to have originated in Ireland, where at the height of the epidemic there were more than 700 000 cases in a population of six million. The English epidemics reached their peak in 1816-19.

During the eighteenth century, typhus became known as "Ship Fever"; together with scurvy, it was one of the most serious scourges of the Royal Navy. It spread from the ships to the shore-based hospitals, thence to the towns and country. At this time, the physician to the naval hospital at Haslar, near Portsmouth, was an enlightened man, named Lind. He did much to overcome scurvy, by devising ways of preserving fruit juices and vegetables during long voyages; he earned popularity for his methods by recommending also garlic-flavoured rum in generous amounts. He also had the absurd (!) idea that typhus was something to do with bedding and clothing, and he took steps to have them cleansed and to a certain extent sterilised; he insisted furthermore on all hospital staff changing their clothes, when they entered or left hospital. Although unaware of the importance of the louse in transmission of typhus, he must have saved many lives by these means.

By the middle of the nineteenth century, it had at last dawned on doctors — and more important on governments and local authorities — that man cannot survive in health in crowded cities, unless provided with pure water in sufficient quantity and with adequate methods for sewage disposal. When hygiene was improved, typhus disappeared, though still prevalent in eastern Europe and Ireland. In the American Civil War typhus was unimportant, though there were 186 000 deaths from disease as against 93 000 battle casualties. In European wars of this time also typhus played no significant part. Yet the disease was smouldering on in Ireland, America and eastern Europe. It was not until 1909 that Charles Nicolle showed that typhus was transmitted from man to man by lice, and at last the simple piece of information was available by which so many lives could have been saved and so much suffering avoided. Even so, during the First World War, 1914-18, typhus flourished on the eastern front. It first appeared in the victorious Serbian army in November 1914. In six months 150 000 persons died in addition to half of the 60 000 Austrian prisoners; of the 400 doctors in the country, 126 died. Had the Austrians counter-attacked at this time, they would have met with no resistance and the course of the war would have been altered.

Typhus was kept from appearing on the western front by strict sanitary measures adopted by both sides. The lessons of Charles Nicolle's discovery had been learned. For the first time in hundreds of years, typhus played no part in military decisions. The disease was absent from the Russian front until the Russian collapse and the breakdown of organised government, which followed the revolution and civil war. In 1916 typhus spread across Russia uninhibited, and it is believed that as many as three million deaths occurred; there were more than twenty five million cases, as is said, so surely many more deaths must have taken place. Epidemics also occurred in Poland, Roumania, Lithuania and the near east.

None, other than the grim story of typhus, can better illustrate the lessons we are seeking to learn from this study. It is the story of how an insignificant disease of rodents became adapted to man living under changed ecological circumstances, with results that were not only disastrous but decisive in many areas of history. We must now study those rickettsioses other than typhus, which are important as zoonoses. None has caused the same widespread effects as typhus, but some of them are none the less important. Table 8 gives a classification of the rickettsial diseases from which man suffers.

TABLE 8
Rickettsial diseases which affect man

Group I — Louse-Borne

Epidemic Typhus. Brill's Disease. Trench Fever etc. *Rickettsia prowazeki*. Affects man alone. Transmitted by human lice (*Pediculus humanus*).

Group II — Flea-Borne

Endemic (Murine) Typhus. *R. mooseri*. A disease of rats and mice. Transmitted to man by rat or mouse fleas, and then by human lice.

Group III — Tick-Borne

Rocky Mountain Spotted Fever and similar infections. Tick Typhus (Boutonneuse Fever). *R. rickettsii* and *R. conorii*. Natural diseases of rabbits, rodents and dogs. Transmitted by various tick species.

Group IV — Mite-Borne

Tsutsugamushi Disease, Scrub Typhus. *R. tsutsugamushi*. Natural hosts, Field Rats and perhaps other small rodents. Transmitted by harvest mites (larvae of species of trombiculid mites).
Rickettsial Pox. *R. akari*. Natural hosts, house mouse in USA and rats in USSR. Transmitted by the rodent mite *Allodermanyssus sanguineus*.

Group V — Q Fever

Q Fever. *Coxiella burneti*. Natural hosts, many wild species including wild rodents, marsupials and domestic farm stock. Transmitted by ticks, but also by air, milk and by contact with organs of infected animals.

Rocky Mountain Spotted Fever

Of the tick-borne rickettsioses, the most important is Rocky Mountain Spotted Fever, which occurs in its most severe form to the west of the Rocky Mountains in the United States; to the east of the mountains, it is more sporadic and less severe. Cases sometimes occur also in other parts of the USA, in the Rocky Mountains regions of Canada, Mexico, Brazil, Columbia and Panama. It is caused by *Rickettsia rickettsii*, the original rickettsia to be described by Ricketts (1906, 1907, 1909). It is transmitted by the wood tick, *Dermacentor andersoni*, in western Montana and by other ticks elsewhere. Ticks are infected at all stages of development and the pathogen can pass through the egg to the next generation. Reservoir animals are small wild rodents. Though some cases are mild, Rocky Mountain Spotted Fever is a dangerous disease with mortality reaching 40% of cases. The symptoms resemble those of epidemic typhus, but the incubation period is shorter, the fever lasts longer and the exanthemata occur at different sites. The rash starts within the 2-4 days, beginning on the ankles and wrists and spreading over the entire body.

Tick Typhus (*Fièvre boutonneuse*)

A similar, but milder, form of Spotted Fever occurs in Mediterranean countries, Africa (from Tunis to South Africa) and in Australia. This form of the disease is caused by *R. conorii* and is known by various names, such as Tick Typhus, Fièvre boutonneuse and others. The disease is endemic in small rodents, but affects also dogs, which are often the vehicle of transmission to man through dog ticks. The transmitting agents are various species of ticks especially the dog tick, *Rhiphicephalus sanguineus*. There is complete cross immunity between *R. rickettsii* and *R. conorii*. In Australia, sera positive to *R. conorii* have been found in some marsupials, bandicoot and opossum. Similar diseases occur also in India and the USSR. These diseases are far less severe than Rocky Mountain Spotted Fever and recovery is rapid. The site of the infected tick bite is marked in most cases by a small ulcer.

Scrub Typhus (*Tsutsugamushi Disease*)

The mite-borne rickettsioses are confined to Japan and the Pacific area, where scrub typhus or tsutsugamushi disease is prevalent. Scrub typhus caused trouble during World War II in the Pacific Zone among allied troops stationed in the Pacific islands, and in parts of China, Burma, Assam, India and Malaya; there were some 18 000 cases with death rates varying from 0·6% to 35%; it was eventually controlled by the use of sulpha drugs and antibiotics. The natural reservoir of scrub typhus is the small rodent, *Microtus montebelloi*, and it is transmitted by a harvest mite, *Trombicula akamushi*; the infecting agent is named

R. tsutsugamushi. Symptoms occur suddenly after an incubation period of 10-14 days with fever, headache, enlargement of lymph nodes and a primary ulcer. The rash develops between 5 and 8 days on the body surfaces and spreads to the arms and legs.

Rickettsial Pox

The second member of the mite-borne rickettsial diseases was described in New York as recently as 1946; it is known as rickettsial pox, because in the late stages the exanthemata develop into vesicles. It is a disease of house mice in the USA, but has also been described in the USSR where rats are infected. It is caused by *R. akari*, and transmitted by a mite parasitic on house mice, *Allodermanyssus sanguineus.* The disease resembles a mild form of endemic typhus with fever, chills, severe headache, pain in the back and a vesicular lesion at the site of the bite. The vesicles, which develop from the maculo-papular rash, disappear without scarification. No deaths have occurred from the disease and recovery is uneventful. The rickettsia is related to *R. conorii* rather than *R. tsutsugamushi.*

Q Fever

The last of the rickettsioses, which must be considered as a zoonosis, is the strange and mysterious disease known as Q Fever, because for so many years it posed a question mark. It is caused by the rickettsial organism known as *Coxiella burneti*, which is given a separate genus in the rickettsial group. Except for Q Fever, the typhus fevers, though varying greatly in severity, all show similar characteristics of symptomatology and transmission by arthropod vectors. Not only are the symptoms of Q Fever uncharacteristic of rickettsioses, but transmission usually occurs other than by intermediate hosts. Its distribution is worldwide, and the organism is found as a harmless commensal in a great range of wild and domestic animals including birds, and in many genera of ticks. It can be spread by these ticks, but is also present in the organs of animals (udder, spleen, liver and kidneys), in the milk, in the placenta and in expired air. Infection in man is usually contracted from contact with animal organs, from urine or faeces, by drinking infected milk or by inhalation.

In domestic animals, coxiella infection is symptomless; in man it causes severe disease with a low mortality except in elderly persons. Q Fever occurs endemically or in local epidemics, affecting chiefly persons working with animals, especially farmers and slaughterhouse workers. The disease caused is a pneumonitis, the typical exanthemata of the typhus fevers being absent. In the late stages, encephalitis may develop. Diagnosis is difficult because of the lack of characteristic symptoms, and it may be overlooked as a cause of pneumonia without laboratory tests.

With this brief account of Q Fever we can leave the rickettsioses. Fuller accounts will be found of typhus and Q fevers in medical textbooks. Here we have learned how a fairly unimportant group of diseases affecting rodents and other animals has evolved pathogens for the human race, some of which are severe and dangerous and are associated with changes of human ecology including, as with syphilis, the wearing of clothes. Epidemic typhus is perhaps the newest of the specifically "new diseases" of man, except for the influenzas which continually recur in "new" form.

CHAPTER 8

Bacterial and Fungal Zoonoses

Introduction

We have already considered some important bacterial diseases, such as plague, syphilis and cholera, and we have noted that man during his urbanised span of life has acquired others that are group specific to him and density dependent. Such are the typhoid and paratyphoid salmonellae and the shigellae of acute bacillary dysentery. No attempt will be made to discuss all the bacterial diseases, which are zoonoses of man. In pursuance of the general theme of this book, we shall concentrate on the enteric diseases and tuberculosis, which have been most important to the health and happiness of urbanised man and which have in some way affected man's history or his habits. It will be convenient here to study the conditions of life in cities, so as to see why such diseases assumed such importance to human welfare. The reasons were the lack of the most elementary knowledge of methods of hygiene and, indeed, indifference to them.

Hygiene in Cities

Cities in earliest times rarely exceeded 10 000 to 20 000 inhabitants, and they were mostly based on agricultural communities. In some early cities, such as the Minoan and even those of Mesopotamia, excreta were removed in primitive water-borne systems or in pits lined with clay latrine pipes. These may have been adequate, provided that the population numbers did not become too high. In other cities, the excreta were removed and used to manure the crops; these practices are today viewed with misgiving for fear that food crops will be contaminated with enteric pathogens. Such dangers appear to be greatly exaggerated, and to this day a great many communities do successfully use human as well as animal manure, thus returning valuable residues to the soil. In cities, such as London, enteric diseases did not become a serious problem so long as night soil systems of sewage disposal were in use and adequate for the level of population. These problems and the development of sewage have been well reviewed by Sir Cedric Stanton Hicks (1975).

Large cities began to be built in Grecian times after the Alexandrine conquests in the second century B.C. Under the Ptolemies, Alexandria and other cities grew to over 100 000 population and this was followed in other parts of the Greek world. In Roman times many more cities, including Rome herself, acquired considerable populations. The Romans brought water to their cities in their great aqueducts, marvels of engineering at the time. Sewage was removed in sewers or "cloacae" from latrines flushed by buckets of water to the rivers and discharged into the sea. The Tiber must have been greatly polluted; indeed, such was the accumulation of silt and effluent that the city port of Ostia at its mouth became buried to a depth of twelve feet and is only now being excavated. However, the water was not used for domestic purposes, so that domestic water and sewage were kept apart unlike European cities in the Middle Ages.

In mediaeval times, towns were small for the most part until after the Black Death, when there was a movement of population away from the country. From then on conditions became progressively worse until the middle of the nineteenth century; those in London were probably typical of what occurred in most mediaeval towns. In the twelfth century each dwelling had a refuse pit, which was emptied by "nightmen" who carried the garbage and sewage to lay stalls outside the city walls. The peasants emptied the middens and carried the material to their fields for use as manure. The streets were cobbled and provided with a central channel to carry off rainwater and household slops. Householders were required to keep clean the pavement and channel in front of their dwellings; the piles of dirt were removed by men called "muck-rakers".

Such arrangements could work satisfactorily in small towns, but were inadequate for a town the size of London. There a great many latrines were built overhanging the river Thames, not then confined within orderly embankments so that much of the river verge consisted of mud flats. The Wallbrook too was lined by a long street of latrines. Ideal conditions were created for the dissemination of pathogens and the stench was truly fearful. Indeed, by the year 1307 the smell from the Fleet River had become so intolerable that a Royal Commission was appointed to seek means of purifying it. However, it was not until 1531-43 and 1601 that regulations were enacted for sewage disposal to be made two miles outside the inner city limits. Even so, by the year 1800 conditions were little, if any, better. As a result of the earlier regulations sewage was being collected in cesspools, and storm water was carried by conduits into the Thames; vegetable garbage was consigned to garbage heaps in the back yards. Latrines were constructed over the cesspools, which were emptied by the nightmen; the garbage was collected by the garbage men. These arrangements were reasonably satisfactory until the invention of the water closet in 1810.

The new invention — the Minoans had invented it three thousand years before — may be a great, if wasteful, blessing in our time. At the beginning of the nineteenth century it put the clock back five hundred years. The death rate reached alarming proportions and was enhanced as the Industrial Revolution got into its stride; the population increased and conditions of overcrowding and filth generally were intensified. In order to accommodate a water-borne sewage system, the cesspools of houses so equipped were linked by open channels to the conduits which formerly only carried stormwater; sewage was again emptied into the Thames. At low tide, it was deposited on the mud flats as in years gone by. The problem was quickly realised and no less than ten Boards of Commissioners of Sewers, each acting independently of the others, were appointed to overcome the problem. Confusion reigned supreme. For example, the Holborn and Finsbury conduits were enlarged while those of the City of London further down the system were not, so that after every heavy rainstorm the houses nearer the river were inundated with sewage. At the same time, there remained a goodly number of cesspits in parts of the city which had not been connected to the sewers, although provided with water closets. These were mostly in Cheapside and Leadenhall Street, where the contents percolated into gravel beds from which domestic water was drawn.

Numerous excellent schemes were put forward to deal with the problem but nothing was done until 1848, either because the Boards concerned were powerless to act, or they disagreed, or parliament refused to appropriate the necessary funds. However, in that year 200 000 cesspits were abolished, and pipe sewers were connected to all houses having water closets. The new sewers emptied raw sewage into the Ravensbourne, the Lee River and the Thames. During slack tide at high water, the solids were deposited on the mud; the rising tide blocked many of the sewer outlets; and the falling tide left behind the jetsam. Conditions were even worse than before. Supplies of domestic water had become contaminated, vermin had multiplied, disease was rampant and the stench was unholy in all parts of London in proximity to the river Thames and its tributaries. Cholera had been introduced from eastern countries and was more or less endemic with especially severe outbreaks in 1832 and 1854; the latter outbreak alone claimed 11 000 victims. In 1855, the stench from the Thames mudflats became so intolerable that the window blinds of the Houses of Parliament were soaked daily with phenol in an attempt to combat it. Not until 1858 was a comprehensive and satisfactory system of sewage disposal put into effect. It had taken more than 500 years for the inhabitants of one of the world's greatest cities to solve the problems of sewage disposal in a way that was adequate to protect the health of the people. Even so, no fully satisfactory solution had been found, or has yet been found, because the fertility of the town wastes was discharged into the rivers and seas instead of being returned to the land. Meanwhile, enormous sums are spent by farmers in importing fertilisers.

In many large cities in the so-called underdeveloped countries, conditions are still no better than those described above. Man lives on his own dung heap; the water he drinks is contaminated; flies breed in millions and carry infection to the food; women die of puerperal sepsis; and the infants do not survive the first few days of life. Infection is harboured in rats and mice and birds, which provide a ready focus from which the flames can be stoked if the fires of disease tend to die down. In these conditions, the human race is degraded; life is cheap and short. Even amongst those that survive, few are fit and well; they are carriers of salmonellae and shigellae, and they are exposed to recurrent illnesses derived from the vermin which infest their cities, such as leptospirosis (Weil's disease) from the rats.

Many overcrowded cities such as these also support large populations of nondescript domestic animals used for food and transport, horses, asses, mules, cattle, sheep, goats and buffalos. Glanders is common in the equine stock, a disease caused by the bacterium, *Pfeiferella mallei*, to which man is very susceptible and which usually proves fatal. The cattle and other ruminants are chronically infected with paratyphoid salmonellae, brucellosis, streptococci and other infections, including tuberculosis. The dangers are enhanced because of overcrowding and a low level of nutrition, common in such situations. The bustling and seemingly thriving scene in a middle or far-eastern bazaar gives little or no indication of the true state of affairs. The visitor finds difficulty in making his way through the apparently healthy, if odoriferous, masses of humanity. He is lucky, however, if he survives for long even in the best hotels without contracting some sewage-borne enteric disease, such as that commonly known as "gyppy tummy". Enquiry at the hospitals will show that few patients are treated for enteric infections, and the resident bacteriologist will explain that the entire population is chronically infected with shigellae and salmonellae and that no account is taken of them. A little research into the mortality statistics, of death at childbirth, of infant mortality and even of life expectation for adults, will reveal a situation he may regard as shocking. However, this is the same situation that prevailed in London and other such cities a mere hundred years ago.

Enteric Diseases

In conditions such as these the incidence of enteric diseases is universal, caused by salmonellae, shigellae and other organisms such as *Proteus spp.*, responsible for infantile diarrhoeas. Most of the adult population will be carriers of some pathogenic organisms, from whom infection will be transmitted during the course of food preparation; animal foods will be largely contaminated. Some children, who become infected early in life, will die. When some of the more serious strains of enteric organisms appear, there will be outbreaks of typhoid or paratyphoid, acute bacillary dysentery or cholera, which will be responsible for deaths amongst the adult population also. It is impossible to assess what has been the influence of these chronic afflictions on human society throughout the ages. They are less spectacular than those of the pandemic and epidemic diseases, but no less insidious. In modern society, as exemplified by the western world, enteric infections have again appeared as a major problem, not because of insanitary conditions in cities and townships but because of newer feeding habits, as will be explained. Meanwhile, let us study the natural history of the salmonelloses.

The Salmonelloses

The salmonellae, which infect man, fall into two groups:— (i) *Salmonella typhosa* which causes true typhoid, and *S. paratyphosa* A, B and C which cause paratyphoid; (ii) other salmonellae which are pathogenic both to man and other animals. Typhoid and paratyphoid can only be contracted by direct or indirect man to man contact, though *S. paratyphosa* has been isolated from monkeys and occasionally infects eggs. These serotypes of salmonellae have plainly come into existence by some rearrangement of salmonella antigens during the long years of man's urbanised existence. A distinction can, therefore, be drawn between the more serious salmonelloses of man, which are not today zoonoses though they originally probably were so, and those which are zoonoses. Whereas in days gone by salmonella epidemics are likely to have been acquired from food or water contaminated from a human source, today the increasingly frequent episodes are mostly contracted from animal sources usually due to improper management of pre-cooked foods.

There are some 300 serotypes of the salmonellae, which differ in the possession of three groups of antigens in different combinations, the flagellar or H antigens, the somatic or O antigens and the superficial "virulence" or Vi antigens. These differences determine the range of animals which may become infected, and the nature and virulence of the infection. Salmonellae, unlike the shigellae, can survive for long periods in moist soil or vegetable material, can infect a wide range of animals and also eggs. Some cold-blooded vertebrates, particularly snakes and tortoises, commonly harbour symptomless infections; tortoises have been responsible for serious outbreaks of salmonellosis in children (*vide* Reichenbach-Klinke and Elkan, 1965). Infections may be of four types: — (i) acute; (ii) chronic; (iii) transitory and symptomless; (iv) the enduring symptomless carrier state. Foci of infection are thus constantly present in nature, especially in rodents and birds. For example, I (unpublished data) examined the bodies of sparrows and starlings, shot at the London Zoo for purposes of study, and found an incidence of infection with *S. typhimurium* as high as 10%; all the infected birds showed some degree of enteritis.

Sources of infection such as these are likely to be of greater primary importance to domestic or captive wild animals than to man, since human food is usually well protected from contamination with avian or rodent faeces. The main source of human infection (*vide* Chapter 13) arises from the consumption of infected meat or meat offals, especially poultry, giving a disease cycle: — wild bird or rodent ⟶ domestic bird or other animal ⟶ man. Alternatively, some domestic animals such as calves become infected with salmonella serotypes characteristic of the species. Again infection may be caused either by produce from an infected animal or from meat that has become contaminated subsequent to slaughter. Another source of infection lies in eggs or egg products, duck eggs being especially dangerous. Dried eggs imported from far eastern countries are widely used in the making of cheap cakes and artificial cream, and are a common source of infection. On one occasion, I traced an outbreak of salmonellosis in parrots to dried egg mixed with the bird seed. In man, the infecting dose of animal salmonellae needs to be relatively large to cause severe clinical symptoms. The reason why such dangers lurk in inadequate refrigeration and reheating of food and maintenance for any length of time at non-sterilising temperatures is that in such conditions a relatively low level of infection becomes massive.

Animal infections with salmonellae are well reviewed by van der Hoeden (1964); they are common in all parts of the world. In cattle they are most commonly caused by *S. dublin*, occasionally by *S. typhimurium*. Veal calves usually become infected towards the end of the first week of life; they suffer from septicaemia, enteritis and pneumonia. Adult cattle suffer from high temperature and profuse diarrhoea. Following recovery, adult cattle frequently become carriers and excrete salmonellae in the faeces; this is unusual in calves. In small ruminants salmonellosis is less common than in cattle, though goats may be infected with *S. dublin* and sheep with *S. typhimurium*. Pigs are frequently infected with a serotype of their own, *S. cholerae-suis*, which has little pathogenicity for man; they can, however, harbour a number of other serotypes, and latent infections in apparently healthy pigs may reach 25%. In dogs and cats, infection with *S. typhimurium* is common and may pass infection to those who handle them. Like pigs, poultry including chickens, ducks, geese and turkeys, have their own pathogenic serotypes in *S. gallinarum* and *S. pullorum*, which are serologically identical. In addition, they can harbour a wide variety of serotypes. Today probably the commonest source of human salmonelloses lies in intensively reared poultry or poultry products, including eggs.

Shigelloses

Unlike the salmonellae, the shigellae have a limited host range. In countries such as Britain, acute bacillary dysentery caused by *Shigella dysenteriae* is extremely rare; this organism is group specific for man and is a common cause of dysentery in African and Asian countries. One instance is recorded of an outbreak of *Sh. dysenteriae* shigellosis in captive chimpanzees, probably acquired from a human source. Of thirteen chimpanzees, from which *Sh. dysenteriae* was isolated, ten died of acute enteritis (Fiennes, 1967). However, in Britain dysenteries due to the *Sh. flexneri* Group, *Sh. sonnei* and *Sh. schmidtii* are annual events; their origin is not clear, probably from persons who are carriers. There is no known animal host which can act as a reservoir of infection apart from simian primates. Monkeys are often seriously affected by shigellosis, usually due to *Sh. flexneri*, and they often die as a result. Frequently, they may be carriers suffering no ill effects or periodic spells of diarrhoea or dysentery. In such cases, it is often extremely difficult to detect infection from faecal cultures, even in monkeys which are sick or die from the disease. At the London Zoo we often found the only means of diagnosis was by the detection of shigella antigens in *Proteus*, which had acquired them by antigen exchange. I have found also that in monkeys the chief seat of infection is in the small intestine, not in the large bowel as in man; this may account for the difficulty of isolating shigellae in faecal cultures. Monkeys that are carriers often escape detection during the routine screening customary for newly acquired animals, and they can be a source of danger both to human beings and to other monkeys long after their quarantine period is over. The dangers for man are discussed at greater length in Chapter 11.

Enteric Disease as a Modern Problem

Enteric diseases, as seen above, are again on the increase in western communities. Some specific incidents, which highlight the dangers, are quoted in Chapter 13. The trouble lies with imported — as with eggs — and pre-packaged foods, deep-freezes and refrigerators, and the food-warming cabinet. In the United States, drugstore feeding has been a national habit for a long time past. In most drug stores and similar places where light meals are served, the food is freshly cooked behind the counter within sight of the customer. Food is, therefore, not normally kept for long periods in warming cabinets; for this reason few instances are recorded of illnesses acquired in these establishments. In Britain, on the other hand, a great many public houses offer meat pies, sausage rolls, cornish pasties and other delicacies, which are placed during the morning in warming cabinets and may not be consumed until some hours later. Regulations prescribe a pasteurising temperature for warming cabinets, but they are continually opened and it is virtually impossible for the temperature to be maintained at a safe level. These cabinets, as often as not, serve as bacteriological incubators; a single salmonella in the original pie will have become billions before it is consumed. The same remarks apply with equal force to the "take-away" meal. In the United States, the greatest trouble is experienced at receptions and outdoor functions, where food is kept hot in the same way or the ambient temperature is high enough to have the same effect. Such outbreaks have often been traced to imported foods, especially from South America, which have been kept frozen. The effect of the freezing is to preserve contaminants in the original food, rather than to destroy them, and to prevent the food from becoming obviously putrid. Another common source of infection in the United States arises from the common practice of home canning. The source of these infections lies predominantly in meat, but vegetables, tomatoes, mushrooms, ice cream and other products have been incriminated. The source of such infections is usually to be sought in contamination of foods with rodent or bird excreta, and they are, therefore, indirect zoonoses. Apart from the usual enteric organisms, another pathogen has become important in recent times, *Yersinia pseudotuberculosis*, the causal organism of pseudotuberculosis. The disease has in the past fifteen years become a nuisance in zoos because of contamination of the food in cages with bird or rodent droppings.

British housewives are aggrieved, because European Common Market rules decree that poultry, including turkeys, must be packaged and deep frozen, whereas they prefer to buy their birds farm fresh over the counter. This regulation has obviously been introduced in the sacred name of hygiene in order to ensure a healthier and purer product. However, research has shown that the incidence of contamination with salmonellae is significantly higher in the frozen product, showing that there are dangers in the packaging and freezing process.

Other Bacterial Pathogens

Before passing to tuberculosis, some other bacterial pathogens which have acquired importance in crowded communities will be considered. In remote times before man congregated in cities, there will have been problems of infectious disease, but they are likely to have been sporadic and to have affected individuals rather than communities. The wildlife hunted by man, and the rodents and birds which shared his habitat, carry pathogens from which man may suffer. Many species of *Lepstospira* and *Listeria* are carried by grazing animals and by rodents. *Brucella* of different species are carried by grazing animals, including reindeer, and pigs. Enteric diseases could have been acquired from rodents and birds, or from eating putrid meat in times of famine. Pasture contaminants, such as anthrax, tetanus and gas gangrene, could be acquired from wound contamination with infected soil; man's close association with horses in Magdalenian times would provide dangers from tetanus. It is not to be supposed, however, that more than a few casualties would occur from such causes, mostly in the younger members of the tribe. That casualties could be higher during, say, the lemming migrations, is possible; these animals are normally carriers of *Pasteurella tularensis*, the cause of a serious and often fatal disease of man tularaemia. Ancient man could also have acquired anthrax as a result of his extensive use of animal skins for clothing and other purposes. However, without large concentrations of stock on the land, this disease is unlikely to have been widespread.

A number of diseases have acquired greater significance in post-glacial times. Let us consider one, which may have had a subtle influence on the course of history and has, in any case, caused much suffering and distress, namely Malta Fever.

Malta Fever

In the truly appalling conditions, which prevailed in mediaeval cities, many chronic diseases of bacterial origin must have been rife in addition to those already discussed, though precise records are lacking. Consumption of milk must have been particularly dangerous. One would suppose that both brucellosis and tuberculosis were transmitted by it. Brucellosis caused by *Brucella abortus* acquired from drinking cow's milk is an unpleasant disease. Malta Fever, caused by *Brucella melitensis*, acquired from drinking goats' milk is not only unpleasant but also dangerous causing numerous deaths. It can also cause lifelong ill health with recurrent and debilitating fevers, Undulant Fever. Goats' milk was widely consumed in Mediterranean countries, and a great many people became chronically infected with Malta Fever. The cause was determined by Sir David Bruce, after whom the brucella organisms were named. It is little known that one chronic sufferer was the French emperor, Napoleon Bonaparte. For all his life he suffered from a mysterious disease which caused fevers at intervals. So concerned was he about this that he gave instructions that an autopsy was to be made on his body after his death, in the hope that a diagnosis could be made and his sons given suitable treatment if also affected.

One occasion, when the emperor suffered symptoms, was at the battle of Waterloo and it is conjectured that, with the advantage on his side, the French might have emerged from the battle victorious, but for the commander being acutely sick at the time. Much has been made of the autopsy results on the emperor's body. Lethal amounts of arsenic were present in Napoleon's liver, nails and hair, and the British Governor of St. Helena has been accused of having him poisoned. The evident truth is that Napoleon was an addicted arsenic eater and may have found that arsenic gave some alleviation of his symptoms. The truth was not made known until many years later in the 1930s. A portion of the emperor's large intestine had been preserved at the Royal College of Surgeons in London. This was examined histologically by the well known British surgeon Lord Moynihan, who gave a lecture in Edinburgh which I attended as a student. Lord Moynihan gave a positive diagnosis of Malta Fever. Since the histology of Malta Fever is uniquely characteristic, the diagnosis cannot be doubted and the symptoms of recurrent fevers are consistent with it. It is surprising that this important fact of history is so little known that the facts surrounding Napoleon's death are still disputed. What, one may ask, would have been the consequences to history of a French victory at Waterloo?

Tuberculosis

Amongst the many diseases rife in cities from mediaeval times onwards, none had more far-reaching or distressing effects than tuberculosis (phthisis, consumption). An excellent review is given by Burnet (1962). Tuberculosis has indeed been the scourge of urbanised man until after the Second World War, when drugs were discovered which were able to cure it. Until then, whole hospitals and clinics were devoted to nothing but tuberculous patients; today they are available to admit patients with other forms of disease. At the same time, the cattle populations of Britain and other countries, formerly riddled with tuberculosis, have been rid of the scourge. The basis of eradication from cattle has been a well organised campaign to create tuberculosis free areas by use of the tuberculin test and slaughter of all reactors; such areas were linked up over the whole country. Drugs and treatment were not used.

We have seen that leprosy and tuberculosis, diseases caused by allied acid-fast organisms, are antagonistic to each other and that tuberculosis displaced leprosy once population concentrations became high (Cockburn, 1963). Tuberculosis is, therefore, a disease of comparatively recent times, and it shows a changing pattern of pathogenesis, which is both instructive and interesting. In man, the disease is caused either by the human bacillus, *Mycobacterium tuberculosis hominis*, or by the related bovine bacillus, *M. t. bovis*. There are many other strains of tubercle bacilli, which cause tuberculosis in fishes, snakes and virtually all vertebrate species, including birds. Avian type bacilli sometimes cause tuberculosis in man and other primates, and in some other mammalian species. The human and bovine strains are only distinguishable from each other by laboratory methods. All tubercle bacilli possess waxy cell coverings, which render them slow to multiply and relatively impervious to the body defences and to most drugs. They are spoken of as acid fast, because certain red dyes, such as carbol fuchsin, can be fixed in the waxy membrane by heat and cannot be removed by acid. The true tubercle bacilli, as opposed to most other acid fast bacilli, are also alcohol and alkali fast. The human and bovine strains differ in their infectivity for laboratory animals, of which those most commonly used to differentiate them are guinea pigs and rabbits. When working at the London Zoo as pathologist, I also found means to differentiate them in artificial culture media, because the use of laboratory animals was not permitted there; these methods I found to be reasonably reliable and quicker than using animals. The method used is summarised under:

A large quantity of tissues or faeces was incubated overnight with caustic alkali (antiformin or caustic potash). Next day the well digested mixture was centrifuged and the deposit stained and examined for acid-fast organisms. Further material, pH adjusted, was seeded on to Loewenstein's or a modified Dubos medium. In the Dubos medium tubercle bacilli, if present, would grow in about eight days, in the Loewenstein in 15 days. The human and bovine strains were differentiated by subculturing on media containing glycerine. *M. t. bovis* is dysgonic and grows poorly on such media, whereas *M. t. hominis* is eugonic and grows well. This technique has been improved since by other workers by using immuno-fluorescent antibody techniques. By these means the existence of pulmonary as well as alimentary tuberculosis can be diagnosed, because the sputum is swallowed by the animals. Even when smears from the digested material are negative, a rare event because it is so highly concentrated, a diagnosis can be reached in 8-15 days and the strain ascertained within a month. Diagnostic methods using animals would take up to three months. The same procedure can identify other pathogens such as lung or skin mites, which are often swallowed.

The two strains of tubercle bacilli also cause different patterns of disease in man and monkeys. The bovine strain is usually more chronic and insidious. The route of infection is usually by ingestion and the primary lesion from which infection spreads is located in the bowel and mesenteric glands. From the primary focus the organisms may spread to other organs, such as the liver, spleen, kidneys, skeleton and joints; if the spine becomes infected, the typical symptoms of Pott's Disease ensue. Lesions of the skeleton, though common with bovine bacilli, are not associated with infections by human bacilli. There is evidence of spinal tuberculosis from ancient Egyptian times onwards, from which it may be inferred that bovine tuberculosis is an ancient disease and that cattle must have been infected.

The human strain of tuberculosis usually enters the body through the respiratory passages. A primary lesion appears in the lungs and from this the disease may spread by the blood and lymphatic systems, and come to infect the pleura, liver, spleen, kidneys and other organs; in children tuberculous meningitis may occur and this is rapidly fatal. There is little evidence of the existence of the human type of disease before about A.D. 1000, and it is evidently a "new" disease; there can be little doubt that it developed from the bovine and thus originated as a zoonosis. It has been one of the most tragic diseases of history often killing the most gifted in early adult life. The Bronte sisters all died young from tuberculosis, while their old parson father lived on giving thanks to God for the lives of his brilliant daughters. The tragedy of early death and separation has been the subject of many literary works, such as "La Dame aux Camélias" by Alexandre Dumas. However, during recorded history tuberculosis has changed markedly in type for reasons, which are of great interest to our argument. The original type of disease is exemplified by that which occurs in children and in Old World, but not New World monkeys (*vide* Fiennes, 1972). This form of the disease is typified by what used to be known as "galloping consumption", usually seen today in children. Progress from the primary lesion of the respiratory tract is rapid and leads to generalised, often miliary, tuberculosis with cavitation of the lungs and wide dissemination of infective bacilli. Spread from the primary focus occurs by four main routes: — (i) by the vascular system; (ii) by the lymphatic system; (iii) by the bronchial tree; (iv) to contiguous organs. The most common sequence of generalisation is lungs, spleen, liver, kidneys and serous membranes. In the lungs are found large coalescing caseous tubercles which lead to consolidation of a great part of the pulmonary tissue, with extensive necrosis and cavitation. Tubercles may be found in any of the thoracic glands, and the disease may spread to the pleura and cause adhesions. The spleen is invariably affected, and infection of the liver is often of the miliary type. The kidneys may be affected with miliary tubercles or large caseous nodules. This is the story of a very serious, acute type of disease, which causes the death of the patient in a few months. In this disease, there is no stage comparable to the chronic isolated disease of adult human beings which may progress slowly to death, or regress to apparent recovery with dangers of subsequent remission.

In recent times, it has been the practice to apply the Mantoux or tuberculin test to children or adults. Mantoux negative children are immunised with BCG vaccine. Amongst the younger generation the percentage of positive reactions has become low, since tuberculosis was controlled by drug therapy. Amongst older people negative results are a rarity, showing that most people have at some time in their lives been assaulted by *M. t. hominis*, but had resisted infection; indeed, persons who have developed active symptoms of tuberculosis are in the minority. Over the centuries, the population has acquired a high degree of immunity to a disease which was formerly of deadly import.

Experience with monkeys may give a clue to one reason for this. The most dreaded catastrophe that can occur in the monkey house at a zoo or a research institute is the introduction of tuberculosis, which may arise from one single animal. This means that the monkey colony is wiped out; not only are very expensive research animals lost, but years of effort or research may be lost also, until a new colony has been developed and the work has been repeated. An infected monkey is not readily detected until the terminal stages of the disease. Initially, there are vague symptoms by no means indicative of tuberculosis; cough may be attributed to lung mite infection, which is almost universal in some species. There is no marked loss of condition, and it is only when the monkey dies rather suddenly after some three to five months, and autopsy is performed, that generalised tuberculous lesions are found. Meanwhile, infection has spread so widely through the colony that it cannot be eradicated; Mantoux negative handlers are at considerable risk. Treatment of monkeys with drugs is less efficacious than in human beings and, except for very valuable animals which can be isolated, is contraindicated for fear of relapses. For these reasons imported monkeys are subjected to strict regimes of quarantine and tuberculin testing for at least six months. This is what usually happens. However, Russian workers from the Sukhumi Research Centre (Lapin and Yakovleva, 1963) deny that this is always so. They point out that the experience of most workers is confined to shipments of highly stressed animals imported under crowded conditions and introduced to crowded quarantine cages in animal houses, that are often not adequately ventilated. In their experience, the transmission rate amongst monkeys kept in the open air, as at Sukhumi, is low and the disease does not always run the usual fulminating course. In addition amongst monkeys kept in this way and fully acclimatised to their new surroundings, the disease is often much milder and regression occasionally occurs. We see, therefore, in monkeys models of both types of human disease, but optimal conditions of life are necessary if the severer type is to be avoided. This is surely analogous to the position in man during the centuries, when city life was so overcrowded and insanitary.

There is, however, another factor which is of importance to the pathogenesis of tuberculosis, and also to our study of the evolution of a "new" disease. It has already been shown that, amongst today's populations in urbanised countries, many individuals repel tubercle infection without showing recognizable symptoms; other individuals given optimal conditions of climate and plentiful rest in bed make a good recovery and are able to return to normal life. Obviously, therefore, individual resistance factors are involved as well as environmental conditions. It will not be surprising to find that the factors of resistance are genetically determined, and this has been statistically proved by studies in identical and non-identical twins. Burnet (1962) evaluates the situation and reviews the studies made by Kallman and Reisner in New York State in the 1940s. These workers abstracted all cases of tuberculosis in twins from the State registers. The families of these "index" cases were then also studied in relation to the incidence of tuberculosis, not only the co-twin but also father and mother, other children and marriage partners. There were 39 pairs of single egg twins and a much larger number of two egg twins, as is usual. The results are shown in Table 9. Identical twins also showed a close resemblance in the type and progress of the disease. Evidence of the operation of the genetic factor can also be obtained from studies of isolated communities, to which tuberculosis has only recently been

TABLE 9

Incidence of tuberculosis in twins and their relations in New York State in the 1940s (from Burnet, 1962)

Relation to index case	Percentage with tuberculosis
One egg twin	87%
Two egg twin	25·6%
Other brother or sister	25·5%
Marriage partner	7·0%

introduced. For example, statistics show that when tuberculosis was first introduced to Mauritius some hundred years ago it was a deadly fulminating disease, but that in the short space of one hundred years it has come to conform to the European pattern. The same experience is true of American Indians, to whom tuberculosis became a "new" disease within living memory. Over a century or more, tuberculosis has by natural selection eliminated the most susceptible members of the population, leaving a community that is relatively resistant. Tragically many of those eliminated have been the most brilliant.

That disease resistance can have such a powerful effect in the selection of urbanised human communities is a point of first class importance, often overlooked by geneticists. One wonders how many other diseases have operated to modify the human gene pool.

Disease caused by Fungi

There are no mycoses that have great relevance to the theme of this book; however, for the sake of completeness a brief account will be given of those, which have some importance as zoonoses. The conditions mentioned are described in greater detail in textbooks on mycology; an interesting review of the mycoses of simian primates, which has some relevance, is given by al Doory (1972). The mycoses are separated into two groups: — (i) the Superficial Mycoses; (ii) the Deep Mycoses. The former cause diseases of the skin, ringworm, favus, tinea. The latter cause systemic diseases, in which the lungs and other organs are affected; some of them are serious. Members of both groups affect wild and domestic animals as well as man.

The Superficial Mycoses

Fungal pathogens which affect the skin are known as dermatophytes; they belong to three genera: — *Trichophyton*, *Microsporum* and *Epidermophyton*. These fungi have an affinity for keratin and live in the keratinized layers of the skin, in nails, horns, hooves, hairs or feathers. Infection may be widespread and severe, or inapparent. The most important member of the Trichophyton group is *T. mentagrophytes* which infects dogs, cats, horses, guinea pigs, rabbits, chinchillas, muskrats, opossums, foxes, squirrels and probably many other animals. The most important reservoir hosts appear to be domestic animals, and captive and wild rodents. Infection in man is rare and tends to self-cure. *T. rubrum*, on the other hand, an occasional pathogen of dogs, causes more serious disease in man, invades the nails and is difficult to cure. *T. verrucosum*, a pathogen of cattle, horses, sheep, goats and donkeys, causes one of the "tinea" diseases of man with suppurating lesions on the scalp or under the beard. The most serious of the trichophyta to infect man is *T. schonleini*, a pathogen of dogs, cats, rats and mice. The disease caused is Tinea Circinata, which can be serious if neglected. The skin becomes covered with large coalescing lesions accompanied by a general infection of the lymphatic glands, which form abscesses and fistulae. When the lesions become widespread, general health is affected. This infection only occurs amongst persons living in poor hygienic conditions; it must have been widespread in mediaeval times, the primary source of infection being rats and mice.

Of the *Microsporum* group of fungi, *M. audouini* is the cause of Tinea Capitis in children. This occurs in epidemics, suggestive of direct spread from child to child. It is not clear whether it originates in a primary animal focus, though there is some evidence to show that some mammals harbour inapparent infections. *M. canis* is the commonest cause of ringworm in dogs, cats and other small mammals. It affects children, who suffer from suppurative lesions of the skin, infection being usually acquired from a dog or a cat; apparently healthy cats can be carriers of the fungus. *M. gypseum* causes ringworm in cats, dogs, mice, rats, monkeys and man. The organism can live an independent existence in the soil, and it appears likely that animals acquire infection from this source and transfer it to man.

The Deep Mycoses

The Deep Mycoses are caused by fungi, some of which may be commensal in the digestive tract; some of them cause serious disease under certain conditions. They are: — coccidioidomycosis, histoplasmosis, blastomycosis and cryptococcosis.

Coccidioidomycosis is caused by a pathogen of wild rodents, known as *Coccidoides immitis*. It is found only in south western United States, and is transmitted in infected dust carried in the wind from rodent burrows. Infection is by inhalation, and granulomatous lesions appear in the lungs and associated lymph nodes. This is a serious disease, which sometimes becomes generalised and proves fatal. Histoplasmosis, due to *Histoplasma capsulatum*, is likewise acquired by inhalation, and is the counterpart of coccidioidomycosis in the eastern parts of the United States. The fungus is found in caves heavily contaminated with bird droppings, which seem to be the source of infection. It has also been found in soil from abandoned chicken runs. In addition to man, cattle, dogs, cats, horses and wild rodents have been found infected. The source of infection is, however, always contaminated dust, since direct infection between animals or from animal to man never occurs.

The lesions take the form of granulomata of the lungs and lymph glands, accompanied by fever, cough, anorexia and weight loss. Usually spontaneous healing takes place with calcification of the lesions, but sometimes the disease becomes generalised and proves fatal. A particularly serious deep mycosis, which occurs only in North America, is Blastomycosis. The lesions are granulomata and abscesses of the lungs and thoracic lymph nodes; sometimes, the viscera and skin are also affected. It terminates in death. Horses and dogs are also susceptible. The mode of transmission is unknown.

Cryptococcosis, caused by *Torula histolytica* (*Cryptococcus neoformans*), causes a fungal meningitis of man, known as torulosis, and mastitis in cattle. Infection is by inhalation of dust contaminated by pigeon droppings. The fungus remains quiescent in the respiratory passages, but may spread to the meninges by way of the blood at times of lowered health or stress.

A number of other fungal infections, such as candidiasis or aspergillosis, could perhaps be regarded as possible zoonoses, but need not in our context be considered as such. There is an evident theme running through the picture portrayed. A great many of man's fungal infections, especially the dermatophytes, are acquired from his domestic animals which in turn acquire them from wild rodents. Primitive man was probably an occasional sufferer from these diseases, yet they have evidently become of greater importance since animals were brought into domestication. None, however, ranks amongst the most important diseases of civilisation and we have, therefore, passed them over lightly. Nevertheless, certain mycoses have acquired increased importance in recent times, especially those such as *Candida*, which can be acquired from animals but which can also be commensals. *Candida* causes "thrush" in children, but can under certain conditions be a serious pathogen of adults also. As a commensal, it lives in competition with the normal bacterial flora of the mouth and throat. Trouble arises, when these are eliminated by the use of antibiotics for respiratory complaints; in these circumstances, *Candida* may multiply to such an extent as to cause a generalised fatal infection.

In the next chapter we shall deal with the Protozoa, one group of which, the Sporozoa, consists entirely of pathogens with no free-living members. These single-celled organisms differ from the pathogens so far considered, in that they are "eukaryotes", that is to say that they have their chromatin aggregated in definite nuclei, and their metabolic processes are in general similar to those of the Metazoa they parasitize. They are nevertheless a highly successful group of pathogens, which have had an important place in human affairs.

CHAPTER 9

Protozoal Zoonoses

Introduction

The parasitic protozoa are grouped in four Classes: — (i) Mastigophora; (ii) Sarcodina; (iii) Sporozoa; (iv) Ciliata. Except for the Sporozoa, all these Classes consist predominantly of free-living Protozoa which occupy a multitude of habitats (mostly aquatic) and perform useful functions in nature. The Sporozoa, on the other hand, are all obligate parasites. The parasitic Ciliata are confined to the intestinal tract, in which many are commensals and do no harm; only a few are important as pathogens or zoonoses. Amongst the Mastigophora and Sarcodina, there are important pathogens, which infect both animals and man and are zoonotic. As a group, the Sporozoa are of great pathogenic importance, both in their own right and as zoonoses. Both Mastigophora and Sporozoa rely to a great extent on transmission by intermediate hosts. A recent review of the parasitic zoonoses is that by Soulsby (1974).

In this study, we shall consider in detail two groups of diseases, the malarias and the trypanosomiases, because they exemplify yet further the problem of the zoonoses as applied to man living in new ecological circumstances. Meanwhile, this is a convenient place in which to devote some attention to the problems of intermediate hosts and arthropod vectors; they are intimately concerned with the transmission of protozoa and are in some ways as important as the pathogens themselves.

Intermediate Hosts and Vectors

A general review of the problems of intermediate hosts in its more important aspects is given by Fiennes (1972). Amongst the mosquitos, many are important vectors of disease, viral, protozoal and helminthic;

in this way they carry diseases from animals to man and are the essential link in the zoonosis chain. Yet, they show certain specificities, both in the animals on which they feed and in the parasites they are able to harbour. We have encountered this problem in relation to Yellow Fever, in which the maintenance of endemic infection in the monkey populations depends on the presence of mosquitos to act as a virus reservoir, a second species to introduce the primary infection to man, and a third urban species to transmit the infection in human communities. In relation to malaria, the situation is even more complex. Mammalian malarias are transmitted by one genus of mosquito only, Anopheles, though avian malarias are transmitted by culicines. The very closely related sporozoan blood parasite of apes and monkeys, *Hepatocystis*, is not transmitted by mosquitos, but by midges of the genus *Culicoides*. In Africa, *Hepatocystis* is the most important blood sporozoan of primates other than man, malaria being insignificant. The differences of life cycle between the two are so seemingly insignificant, that the requirements of completely different vectors is surprising. In order, to illustrate this point, a brief account will be given of the life histories of the two organisms. For a fuller account, see Voller (1972).

In the malarias, caused by *Plasmodium spp.*, a small needle-like sporozoite is injected into the host by the mosquito, which after a few minutes penetrates a parenchymal liver cell. In this cell a small spherical structure develops, which enlarges over a period of one to two weeks to form a pre-erythrocytic schizont. After one to two weeks more, the schizont ruptures releasing thousands of merozoites which enter the blood stream. The merozoites enter the red blood corpuscles and start a new stage of the life cycle, that of the trophozoite or feeding stage. In the red cells cell division takes place and erythrocytic schizonts are formed containing a further generation of merozoites. The schizont next bursts, destroying the red cell, and the merozoites are released to invade new cells. All the clinical and pathological symptoms of malaria are attributable to the asexual erythrocytic cycle. Some of the merozoites after a few generations develop into gameto-cytes, the sexual forms, instead of into schizonts. The male and female gametocytes are ingested by mosquitos during the course of a blood meal; they then undergo anisogamy, fusion, to form a zygote in the mosquito. The zygotes are motile ookinetes, which move to the stomach wall to form oocysts. The oocysts burst in one or two weeks to produce further infective sporozoites, which pass to the salivary glands.

With *Hepatocystis* the injected sporozoites invade liver cells in the same way, but form very much larger cysts than plasmodia; visible to the naked eye, they are known as merocysts. Many more hepatic

TABLE 10
Transmission of simian malarias

Species	Host	Transmission
I. Tertian malarias		
1) *Plasmodium vivax*	Man	Anopheles spp. (more than 40)
2) *P. schwetzi*	Chimpanzee	
	Gorilla	
	Man (with difficulty)	Unknown. Will not infect *A. gambiae* (stenoxenous)
3) *P. eylesi*	Gibbon	Local Malayan Anopheles
4) *P. jefferyi*	Lar gibbon	Unknown
5) *P. cynomolgi*	Macaques	Anopheles spp. (more than 35) especially *A.*
	M. irus	*balabacensis, A. hackeri, A. elegans, A. kochi*
6) *P. c. bastianellii*	Macaques	Unknown
7) *P. c. cyclopis*	*M. cyclopis*	Unknown
8) *P. c. ceylonensis*	Toque monkeys	
	Grey langurs	Unknown
9) *P. ovale*	Man; chimpanzee experimentally	Unknown; probably *A. gambiae, A. funestus*
10) *P. simium*	Howlers	Probably *A. cruzi*
11) *P. fieldi*	*M. nemestrina*, rhesus experimentally	*A. hackeri, A. balabacensis*
12) *P. simiovale*	*M. sinica*	Unknown
13) *P. gonderi*	Cercopithecus spp.	
	Sooty mangabeys (*Cercocebus fuliginosus*)	Unknown
14) *P. coatneyi*	*M. irus*	*A. hackeri*
15) *P. fragile*	*M. radiata*	Unknown
	M. sinica	
II. Malignant subtertian malarias		
1) *P. falciparum*	Man	Anopheles spp. (more than 60)
2) *P. reichenowi*	Great apes	Unknown
III. Quartan malarias		
1) *P. malariae*	Man	*A. gambiae, A. aconitus,*
	Chimpanzee	*A. annulipes, A. darlingi, A. funestus, A. sacharovi*
2) *P. inui*	*M. mulatta, M. irus, M. nemestrina, M. lasiotis*	*A. hackeri, A. leucosphyrus*
3) *P. shortii*	Toque monkeys	Possibly *A. stephensi*
4) *P. brasilianum*	Saimiri spp., Cebus spp. Alouatta spp. Leontocebus, *Aotus infumatus*, Uakari	Probably *A. neivai*
5) *P. girardi*	Lemur	Unknown
IV. Special groups		
1) *P. pitheci*	Orang-utan	Unknown
2) *P. hylobati*	Gibbon	Unknown
3) *P. youngi*	Gibbon	Unknown
4) *P. knowlesi*	*M. irus* and macaques	
	Presbytis,	*A. hackeri*
	Semnopithecus,	*A. pujutensis*
	Experimentally, baboon which dies, gibbon, *Callithrix*	

merozoites are produced than with plasmodia; they, like plasmodia, invade red blood cells and develop directly into male or female gametocytes but no erythrocytic schizogony takes place. The difference, on the face of it, appears comparatively slight; yet the parasite requires a different vector, has a specialised host range in the lower primates only and is rightly placed by taxonomists in a different genus from the malarias.

Even with the anopheline mosquitos themselves there are peculiar anomalies, which affect their role as potential transmitters of zoonoses. Some plasmodia are euryxenous and can infect a broad range of anopheles; others are stenoxenous infecting only a narrow range. Furthermore, closely related malaria parasites may require entirely different vectors. For example, *Plasmodium vivax* of man can be transmitted by at least forty species of Anopheles; the equivalent *P. schwetzi* of chimpanzees and gorillas will infect none of this range in so far as they have been tried, and the natural vector has yet to be discovered. Similarly, *P. falciparum*, which causes the very serious malignant subtertian malaria of man, can be transmitted by at least sixty species of Anopheles, but it has not been possible to find any vectors of the closely related *P. reichenowi* of the great apes. Table 10 shows the differences between the malarias of man and other primates in respect of hosts and vectors.

The Malarias as Zoonoses

The simian malarias are reviewed in such works as Garnham (1966), Fiennes (1967) and Voller (1972). Evidence as to the infectibility of simian malaria parasites for man, especially in the Far East and South America, formerly gave cause for concern that malaria eradication schemes might be thwarted by reintroduction of simian malarias from jungle sources. This fear led to wide-scale investigations. Accidental transmission of *P. cynomolgi* to man from a monkey had occurred in the laboratory, the infection being naturally acquired by mosquito bite. In the field, two infections of man with *P. knowlesi* had occurred under natural conditions in Malaysia, and one with *P. simium* in Brazil. Such determinations could well be the tip of the iceberg, since precise identification of the parasite in malaria cases might not be made in the absence of experienced malariologists. As a result of laboratory investigations, the following simian malarias have been classified as potential zoonoses:— *P. cynomolgi* (Asia), *P. knowlesi* (Asia), *P. inui* (Asia), *P. schwetzi* resembling *P. ovale* (Africa), *P. rhodaini* (Africa), *P. brasilianum* resembling *P. malariae* (South

America), *P. simium* resembling *P. vivax* (South America). The importance of malaria as a zoonosis has today been largely discounted, because of the small numbers of simian malarias that have been diagnosed in man. This view must be altogether too short-sighted. The virulence and serious consequences of the pathogenic human malarias proclaim them to be "new" diseases, and they can only have been derived from their simian counterparts. It is significant that these malarias, unlike their simian predecessors, are transmitted by a wide range of anopheline mosquitos; the mutation of the parasite would seem therefore to lie more in adaptation to a new intermediate host than to a new secondary host. If this has happened before, it could happen again. Furthermore, it is believed by malariologists that simian malarias in South America were originally derived from human counterparts and thus originated as anthroponoses. If so, then the plasmodia could surely retread the road of infection and again become adapted to man.

The form of malaria parasite, to which man is best adapted is *P. ovale*, the equivalent of the simian *P. schwetzi*. This parasite does not cause malarial symptoms, and its only significance lies in its recognition in blood smears so as to differentiate it from the more harmful plasmodia. *P. ovale* plainly fills the role of man's indigenous, ancestral plasmodium; host and parasite have become fully adapted to each other over many millennia. Man suffers also from three other malarias: — 1. Benign Tertian, caused by *P. vivax*; 2. Quartan, caused by *P. malariae*; and 3. Malignant Subtertian, caused by *P. falciparum*. All three cause acute symptoms of disease. *P. falciparum* is a very dangerous pathogen and is responsible for more human deaths annually than any other; it is almost universally fatal to sufferers when introduced newly to uninfected areas. In endemic areas, it is responsible for a heavy toll of deaths in young persons, commonly 15% or more; it also causes prolonged ill health throughout the early years of life up to an age of 17 or so, interfering with the ability of young people to learn and retarding the mental faculties. In contrast to *P. ovale*, *P. falciparum* is evidently a recently acquired pathogen of man. After recovery, the parasite is eliminated from the body within 18 months; the disease is, therefore, density dependent, because in the absence of sufficient people to maintain infection in the mosquito populations it will disappear. The other three plasmodia of man can be retained in silent form for many years, if not for a lifetime.

Quartan is the least serious of man's pathogenic malarias, and was probably the cause of the agues from which people suffered from time to time in European countries. Benign Tertian is largely a disease of Mediterranean countries; Malignant Subtertian of the tropics. Benign Tertian and Malignant Subtertian are both associated with genetical disorders of the blood, which can of themselves be serious but militate against fatal malarial infections. These disorders, known as Thalassaemia and Sickle-cell Anaemia, are associated with the presence of abnormal haemoglobins, the presence of which can be responsible for serious or fatal disease but which can frustrate the entry of malaria parasites into red cells which carry them. An excellent brief account of thalassaemia is given by Williamson (1977), who believes that the disease is the most common hereditary defect in the world. Some six million persons are affected amongst white and yellow people living in a broad belt from the western Mediterranean through the Middle East to Thailand and Malaysia. Sickle cell anaemia affects chiefly black populations in West African countries. The genetics of the two diseases are entirely different, showing that they have been independently evolved. Those of thalassaemia affect either the alpha or beta globin chains of the haemoglobin molecule, and the nature of the disease differs depending on which chain is affected. In the case of Sickle cell Anaemia, an abnormal haemoglobin, the S haemoglobin, is present in the blood. All children homozygous for the S haemoglobin gene, receiving the gene from both parents, fail to survive; those that are homozygous in the sense that they do not possess S haemoglobin stand a good chance of succumbing to malaria in infancy; those that are heterozygous, that is receive the S gene from one parent only, stand a better chance of survival, because they are partially resistant to malaria. On Mendelian principles, one in four children born will die of sickle-cell anaemia; one in four stand a good chance of dying of malaria; two in four stand a good chance of surviving malarial attacks until they are adult. Though the mechanisms are different, the results are similar with thalassaemia. Nothing could better illustrate the important role of malaria in human ecology in tropical and sub-tropical countries, when population densities are high enough to maintain infection in the intermediate host.

The Origins and Distribution of the Malarias

These genetic changes and the severity of malarial infections show that the pathogenic malarias of man have arisen in remote times from some animal source; one may be reasonably sure that the original source must have been simian. For *P. falciparum*, the only possible source is *P. reichenowi*, the only other malignant sub-tertian parasite, which infects chimpanzees and gorillas; its origins, therefore, were in Africa at a time when the African apes were more numerous and man's hunting activities took him frequently into the forests where they lived. The Benign Tertian and Quartan malarias, as will be seen from the table above, give a greater choice of origin amongst an assortment of monkey species, most of which are Asian. They are likely, therefore, to have originated in the east or far east. That there are three different malarias suggests that there have been three separate occasions on which they have become adapted to man. The conditions for this to occur would be a high concentration of population leading to an increase of anopheles numbers, and perhaps a change of habits of the mosquitos; thirdly, once a number of people was infected with monkey malaria the plasmodium could become adapted to a new vector species and produce a new strain, which was man-dependent instead of monkey-dependent. As we have seen, malariologists suppose that this is how South American monkeys originally acquired their malarias from human sources, so that there is no difficulty in believing that the human malarias arose in the opposite way.

In northern areas, the distribution of anopheles is somewhat irregular. In Britain, for example, they are only found in East Anglia and Hayling Island in Southampton Water. They are found in the Pripet Marshes on the Polish Russian frontier, in low lying areas of the Netherlands, and as a result of land mismanagement in Tuscany and the Pontine Marshes near Rome. In the Netherlands malaria was until recently a serious problem. There exist in Holland two races of *Anopheles maculipennis*, which are morphologically indistinguishable from each other (*vide*, Burnet, 1962). Yet the two races have different habits; the one transmits malaria, the other does not. The transmitter breeds in brackish water, the non-transmitter in fresh water. The transmitter winters on the ceilings of farmhouses; the non-transmitter hibernates and is inactive all winter. When the transmitter takes a blood meal in winter, it can transmit malaria, but there is a long incubation period and the disease does not develop until summer. This story illustrates how the mosquitos are able to adapt themselves to varying circumstances, and how malarial pathogens too may vary in their pathogenesis.

The Importance of Malaria

Malaria is undoubtedly the most important of all endemic infectious diseases. According to estimates, there were in 1930 in India alone some hundred million persons infected, with a death rate running at two million per annum. Its importance, however, extends far beyond the visible results of illness and death. It has been responsible for the devitalization of whole populations. It has deprived young people in backward areas of their capacity to develop intellectually, so that they earn the reputation of being intellectually incompetent. Malaria may well have been a major cause of the decline and fall of the Greek and Roman empires. An epidemic of malaria in Ceylon in 1934 to 1935 was the greatest, since accurate records have been kept; there were 80 000 deaths from two to three million cases. In endemic areas, infants become infected at an early age and are subject to frequent reinfections if they survive. Many die in early life, either directly from malaria or from other infections which attack them because they are debilitated from malaria. Children remain chronically infected until they are some eighteen years of age, and suffer from greatly enlarged spleens. About that age, the spleen regains its normal size, and the patient becomes tolerant of, or resistant to, further infection and apparently healthy. However, if conditions are poor and the population crowded and underfed, malarial symptoms may recur. Over centuries, malaria has operated as the great population regulator. Today, malaria can be controlled, even eradicated, by treatment with drugs and elimination of mosquito breeding by DDT and other insecticides. When this is done, population explosions occur in areas where food may already be in short supply; then further problems of human ecology are posed. Furthermore, when malaria is eradicated, there are ready dangers of its reintroduction at a time in the future, when a new susceptible population has arisen; the results can be disastrous.

In many parts of the world, the extreme menace of malaria has been the direct result of land mismanagement. Such occurred in Italy during imperial Roman times. The situation there has been closely studied over many years by Sir Cedric Stanton Hicks (1975), from whom some excerpts are quoted: —

> The story begins about 800 B.C. with the Etruscans, who appear in history as farmers working the land that they had cleared from the forest surrounding their walled towns, usually perched on some high rock outcrop for defence against other Italic tribes . . . Their chief cities were in Etruria, the region between the Tiber and Pisa, and it is in this region, as well as that immediately south of Rome, that their agricultural skills were so highly developed. The Apennines are very high mountains, and rainstorms are heavy, with resulting torrential runoff. The rolling, soft, volcanic tufa country favoured both erosion and swamp formation on cleared land. This the Etruscans handled with a display of brilliant engineering. They drove diversion tunnels through the sides of valleys and through ridges, creating a veritable network of drainage systems which only recently have been recognised and adequately studied. Part of the coastal region of the Maremma is today drained by the ancient Etruscan system, which, after running west along the coast, empties into the sea through an impressive cutting and tunnel through Monte Argentino. The outlet is cunningly protected from the backthrust of the sea by a breakwater cut out of the solid limestone of the cliff face.
>
> The Etruscans used bronze and then iron ploughshares, and a conservative system of two to three crop rotations adopted and used by the Romans during the early Republican period.

Sir Cedric goes on to explain how the Romans adopted the Etruscan system and farmed the land carefully and well, until the era of conquest. The farms were then sold to wealthy senators and war profiteers. The land was worked by chain gangs of slaves, and "all the patient care of the soil, the manuring, the fallow, the rotations, and the maintenance of drainage and of careful animal husbandry were more and more neglected". By 140 B.C., the Maremma was desolate and uninhabited; Tiberius Gracchus attempted to have the situation rectified, but was opposed by vested interests and assassinated. Under the Empire attempts were made to restore the situation but conditions had deteriorated too far. Both in the Maremma and at the mouth of the Tiber at Ostia malarious marshes had developed, and all attempts to resettle these areas until the present time failed because of the high incidence of malaria in settlers. It is only in very recent times, that some success is being achieved in eradication of malaria and reclaiming valuable agricultural land.

The results of malarial infection on the evolution and history of civilised man have been incalculable. Whole races of mankind have been debilitated by it and genetic interference has occurred, with unknown results. Life expectation has been drastically reduced by it, and the tendency has been for early marriage and child-bearing to be compressed into a shortened breeding life with insufficient intervals between pregnancies. When the limiting factor is removed, rapid breeding continues and population explosion occurs into lands without the capacity to produce enough food. Solution of the malaria problem thus creates new problems of population control, which are equally intractable.

The Trypanosomiases (*Sleeping Sickness*)

The second group of diseases to be discussed under the heading of Protozoal Zoonoses is that of the trypanosomiases, including Sleeping Sickness. Trypanosomes are widespread in nature as a group of blood and tissue parasites, being found in fish, amphibia, reptiles, birds and most orders and species of mammals. Often enough they are non-pathogenic, and it may be difficult to demonstrate their presence in the host. Their relationships with their hosts are complex and the methods by which they are transmitted are very variable indicating that, in spite of their widespread distribution, they may in some hosts be rather recent parasites. The trypanosomal disease of horses known as "dourine" is venereal and transmitted during coitus. Trypanosomes are also transmitted by a wide variety of intermediate hosts in a number of different ways. *Trypanosoma evansi*, which causes the disease of "surra" in camels and horses, is transmitted by biting flies, such as *Tabanus, Haematopota* and *Stomoxys*; the transmission is purely mechanical, infected blood being carried on the fly's proboscis from one animal to another. *T. lewisi*, a harmless parasite of rats, is transmitted by fleas; the parasites are present in the faeces of the flea and are introduced to the system when the faeces are rubbed in by scratching the bite. The so-called monomorphic trypanosomes develop in the gut of tsetse flies being regurgitated into the saliva when a blood meal is taken; in this way they are injected, when the host is bitten. Typical of this group is *T. congolense*, a deadly scourge of cattle in tsetse infested areas of Africa. Trypanosomes of the "salivarian" group, which contains those responsible for Sleeping Sickness of man, develop in the salivary glands of the tsetse flies, and thus show a further step in adaptation to transmission by an intermediate host.

There are two distinct forms of trypanosomiasis from which man suffers, African Trypanosomiasis or Sleeping Sickness caused by *T. brucei gambiense* or *T. b. rhodesiense*, and American Trypanosomiasis or Chagas Disease, caused by *T. cruzi*. The African trypanosomiases have been extensively reviewed by Mulligan (1970). The African trypanosomiases of man occur solely in Africa and are transmitted by tsetse flies (*Glossina spp.*); the American occurs solely in South and Central America and is transmitted by reduviid bugs (*Rhodnius prolixus*) which attack the host when he is asleep at night. There is no sharp demarcation line in Africa between Gambian and Rhodesian Sleeping Sickness. The Gambian is more prevalent in the western and northern parts of the central African belt, especially near rivers and lakes, whereas Rhodesian is more prevalent in south eastern parts such as Rhodesia, the former Portuguese East Africa and Tanzania. Gambian Sleeping Sickness is more chronic and insidious, whereas Rhodesian is usually an acute disease. Nevertheless, the two forms of the disease are caused by strains of an organism, which are morphologicall identical and indistinguishable also from *T. brucei brucei* which infects cattle, dogs, pigs and horses, but only occasionally man.

The great sleeping sickness epidemic hit Uganda in the early years of the twentieth century, a country which had become a British Protectorate in 1894, after some years of missionary endeavour and rule by the British East Africa Company. It is supposed that the disease was newly introduced from West Africa by porters, who had accompanied Henry Stanley on his famous journey up the Congo River in search of Emin Pasha. The southern part of the country is endowed with swampy rivers and lakes, along which the main vectors of Gambian Sleeping Sickness, *Glossina palpalis*, breed in large numbers, feeding mostly on crocodiles and other cold-blooded fauna. Up to this time, the tsetse flies appear to have been uninfected, but once infection was introduced sleeping sickness spread rapidly through the indigenous populations.

The situation was most acute in the Busoga District on the northern shores of Lake Victoria in eastern Uganda. At this time southern Busoga was heavily populated with a prosperous people, living on their shambas of plantains and other crops. Within ten years some 50 000 persons had died, and the surviving population had been moved inland out of harm's way. To this day, the country, well known to the author, is covered by thick secondary forest, in which buffalo and other wildlife abound. It has also become infested with the tsetse fly, *Glossina pallidipes*, which transmits cattle trypanosomiasis, and cannot even be used, therefore, for grazing cattle. So serious was the situation that the Royal Society in London organised its Sleeping Sickness Commission under the direction of Sir David Bruce to investigate its causes. Bruce, born in Australia, received his medical education in Edinburgh and joined the army as a surgeon. He served in Malta, Egypt and South Africa, and was known for his discovery in 1887 of the causative agent (*Brucella melitensis*) of Undulant or Malta Fever. In 1895, he showed that "nagana" of cattle in Zululand was caused by a trypanosome to be named *T. brucei*; in fact it is caused by *T. congolense* and it appears that Bruce mixed up the blood slides he sent to London, so that the wrong trypanosome was named after him. All the same, he was the first to show that trypanosomes could cause serious disease. He was preceded to Uganda by a young Portuguese doctor, Castellani, who had demonstrated the presence of trypanosomes in the blood and spinal fluid of sleeping sickness patients by the time of Bruce's arrival. It was quickly established that they were the cause of the disease, though controversy raged for decades as to whether the credit for the discovery belonged to Bruce, who claimed it, or to Castellani; Bruce maintained that, though Castellani had demonstrated the presence of the trypanosomes, he was unaware of the significance of their presence until he had been enlightened by Bruce. At this time also, a German team was working on sleeping sickness in the then German East Africa, now Tanzania, under a well known medical scientist, Kleine. To Bruce's considerable chagrin, proof of the transmission of sleeping sickness by tsetse flies was achieved first by the Germans, only weeks before it was demonstrated by the team working under Bruce.

Gambian Sleeping Sickness is transmitted predominantly by the riverine and lacustrine tsetse flies, *Glossina palpalis*, whereas Rhodesian Sleeping Sickness is predominantly transmitted by savannah type tsetses, *G. morsitans*. Earlier workers found that, if human populations were removed from an area where Gambian Sleeping Sickness existed, it could after a time be safely repopulated, even though the tsetse flies were not removed. This would indicate that there was no wildlife reservoir of *T. b. gambiense*. The same is not true of *T. b. rhodesiense*, which certainly exists in wild herbivores. This simple position has recently been questioned, because it is said that *G. palpalis* does not normally feed on the wildlife hosts of *brucei* type trypanosomes. The absence of *T. b. gambiense* from wildlife is, therefore, attributed to the feeding habits of the transmitting fly. However, it can be transmitted by other tsetses, so that the dangers exist that a wildlife reservoir could at some time be created, and it is difficult to see why it did not happen at the time of the great epidemic. Today, the trypanosomiases are more readily diagnosed and can be effectively treated. Control is, therefore, possible. Control by eradication of tsetse flies presents problems which have still not been solved in spite of years of intensive research and recourse to the most ingenious stratagems. Enormous areas of tropical Africa are virtually depopulated because of tsetse infestation, which renders them unsuitable for cattle raising. Many peoples in Africa number their wealth by their livestock and are reluctant to settle, where they cannot be kept. In parts of West Africa, Sleeping Sickness appears to have been endemic for centuries and, with other diseases, has no doubt contributed to the slow progress made by the indigenous peoples.

As zoonoses, the African trypanosomiases have evidently arisen from wildlife trypanosomes of the *brucei* group. They are not important diseases of monkeys (Fiennes, 1967). In Serengeti, cryptic infection was found to be as high as 78%, though in Queen Elizabeth Park in Uganda only 11% carried infection. These infections were presumably for the most part *T. b. brucei*, though this could only be determined by infecting human volunteers. Rhodesian Sleeping Sickness which, unlike Gambian, causes a very acute type of disease in man, certainly exists in wildlife reservoirs; it may be a much more recently evolved disease than Gambian, derived from a parent *brucei* strain. In the early stage of Gambian Sleeping Sickness, infection is confined to the blood and lymphatic systems. This is the stage at which the more severe symptoms appear in the Rhodesian Disease, whereas in the Gambian they are usually so mild as in some cases to be inapparent. In the later stage, the nervous system is invaded, and it is only then that the characteristic symptoms of Sleeping Sickness appear and the disease becomes serious and eventually lethal. Some cases have been recorded, in which white men have developed Sleeping Sickness years after leaving Africa. Gambian Sleeping Sickness, while it plainly comes within our definition of "new" diseases, would appear to have infected man for many generations; adaptation of host to parasite and vice versa seems well advanced.

Gambian Sleeping Sickness, then, must have originated as a zoonosis, but today is transmitted solely from man to man through tsetses. Rhodesian Sleeping Sickness, on the other hand, may well reappear from animal reservoirs. Some observers, however, are doubtful whether this actually happens. Onyango *et al* (1966) for example believe that epidemics usually arise when some infected person has entered country infested with the transmitting agent. Another possibility exists, namely that some person may acquire infection with *T. b. brucei*, which could as a result acquire the properties of *T. b. rhodesiense* and be transmitted as such to other persons.

Chagas Disease (South American Trypanosomiasis) is a recognised zoonosis, though some observers believe that the human reservoir is the most important. The most important animal reservoirs are considered to be dogs, cats, armadillos and opossums, though monkeys can carry infection. The infecting triatomid bugs are large creatures, which lay their eggs on palm leaves and the palm thatch of huts. The adults emerge from the palm thatch at night to feed. The bug's faeces are infected, and trypanosomes are introduced to the host when the faeces are rubbed into an abrasion of the skin or into the eye. The trypanosomes do not multiply in the blood like the African trypanosomes, but in the cells of internal organs, especially the heart and other muscles. Death from cardiac failure, arising from degeneration of the cardiac muscle, commonly occurs. Chagas Disease is more acute in children than in adults causing the so-called Parasitic Thyroiditis. Adults suffer from chronic ill health and anaemia. In spite of the extensive researches on it, there is still some mystery surrounding the pathogenesis of Chagas Disease. When on sabbatical leave at the Delta Regional Primate Center, New Orleans, I found a colony of trypanosomes resembling *T. cruzi* in the heart muscles of a gibbon (unpublished data); the gibbon, an east Asian ape, had never been within the Chagas Disease endemic area nor exposed to rhodnius; the origin and nature of the infection is a profound mystery.

Other Protozoal Zoonoses

The malarias and the trypanosomiases are unquestionably the most important of the protozoal zoonoses. There are other sporozoan zoonoses, such as the babesiases which are coming to be recognised as having significance, but need not be discussed in our context. There are other flagellates (Mastigophora), such as *Giardia lamblia*, which are zoonoses and cause mild diseases in man. Amongst the Sarcodina, *Entamoeba histolytica* causes serious and sometimes fatal disease, amoebiasis, in man, and can be acquired from pigs, apes and monkeys. Amongst the ciliates, *Balantidium coli* can also be acquired from pigs, apes and monkeys. We need not dwell on them, but must consider two important zoonoses: — first, the leishmaniases caused by *Leishmania spp.*, which are flagellates; secondly, toxoplasmosis caused by a sporozoan organism, *Toxoplasma gondii.*

The Leishmaniases

The leishmanias are a widespread group of parasites, which are all transmitted by sandflies, *Phlebotomus spp.*; their epidemiology is linked to the life histories of these flies. In the vertebrate host, they are intracellular parasites of the macrophage or reticulo-endothelial system, in which they appear as rounded bodies with distinct nuclei and characteristic rod-shaped kinetoplasts, the Leishman-Donovan bodies. In the intermediate host, they develop flagellated leptomonad forms that lack the characteristic undulating membranes of trypanosomes. Three forms of leishmaniasis are described: —

1. Visceral Leishmaniasis or Kala-Azar caused by *Leishmania donovani.*

2. Cutaneous Leishmaniasis or Oriental Sore caused by *L. tropica.*

3. American Muco-cutaneous Leishmaniasis or Espundia caused by *L. brasiliensis.*

Visceral leishmaniasis develops somewhat different forms in different parts of the world, that is the Mediterranean region, India, China, Central Asia, East Africa and South America. The main symptoms are an irregular, not very high, fever, weakness, emaciation, enlargement of spleen and liver, together with non-specific symptoms such as cough and diarrhoea. Mediterranean Leishmaniasis usually proves fatal within a few months unless treated. Apart from the Mediterranean, one other main form of the disease, the Indian, is recognised, though other forms, such as that encountered in China, are intermediate. The differences between the Mediterranean and Indian forms are of especial importance to the study of zoonoses. The Mediterranean form affects dogs and other carnivores as well as children, whereas the Indian form affects man alone. The Indian form occurs in epidemics depending on man to man transmission by sandflies; the Mediterranean form is sporadic being transmitted from wild or domestic carnivores by the sandflies. It is only in India that *L. donovani* is pathogenic to man alone, demonstrating yet another instance of a pathogen which, in spite of its animal origins, has become solely adapted to man.

L. tropica, the cause of Oriental Sore, causes purely local lesions of the skin; these last for a year or two leaving persistent scars but also immunity to reinfection. The disease, which is carried by some rodents, dogs and cats, occurs in the Mediterranean region, extending through the Near and Middle East into Turkestan and Pakistan. Some isolated foci are present in West Africa and East Asia.

South American Muco-cutaneous Leishmaniasis resembles Oriental Sore, but metastatic lesions occur affecting the mucosa of the mouth and nose, causing rodent ulcers which bite deeply into the tissues and can even cause destruction of the lips or external nares. Wild rodents and carnivores are also affected.

In general, leishmanias parasitize domestic animals and man only secondarily. Their natural hosts are lizards, marsupials, rodents, carnivores, edentates and insectivores. Human infections, *L. donovani* apart, mostly arise at second hand from dogs, which have acquired infection from wild species. Phlebotomus have somewhat exacting requirements for breeding, correct temperature and moisture. Such conditions are provided in rodent and other animal burrows; dogs acquire infection during hunting activities which take them to the burrows. Some workers maintain that the classification of the leishmania is by no means so simple as stated above; for a more detailed account Bray (1974) should be consulted.

Toxoplasmosis

Toxoplasmosis, caused by *Toxoplasma gondii*, is a worldwide zoonosis with no host specificity; any warm-blooded animal or bird can be affected. Although it is a sporozoan, it does not require an intermediate host or vector, in this respect resembling the Coccidia of which it is probably an aberrant member. Toxoplasma are intracellular parasites and virtually any nucleated cell can be parasitized, though reticulo-endothelieal cells are preferred. When introduced into the body, the parasites multiply and spread until they kill the host or immunity is developed. When immunity begins to appear, the parasites form tissue cysts, usually in the brain, less commonly in the heart, skeletal muscles or lungs. The cysts persist for months or years, or even for the lifetime of the host. In man, congenital infection can occur, if a primary infection is contracted during pregnancy; a generalised infection of the foetus results, by which it may be killed; if it survives, the infection becomes localised in the central nervous system. If the infection is acquired at a late stage of pregnancy, the child may show symptoms two to three months after birth. The usual course of infection in man, especially in children, is a low grade hyperpyrexia which may not be detected, together with general malaise, fatigue and sometimes muscle pains. The symptoms resemble those of Glandular Fever (Infectious Mononucleosis) mentioned earlier, and can only be differentiated by serological tests. Sometimes, there are ocular or cerebral symptoms which can be serious; indeed, dogs sometimes develop symptoms which have been mistaken for rabies. Sheep and pigs are commonly infected and the infection can be passed to human hosts in undercooked lamb or pork. However, the main vehicle of infection for man is the cat, involving a disease cycle that is of exceptional interest.

In rodents, toxoplasma are passed congenitally from generation to generation, so that a reservoir exists wherever there are rats and mice. Cats become infected from eating mice; once in the cat the parasite undergoes a development cycle, which is peculiar to the cat and does not occur in any other host animal. The cycle resembles that of Coccidia, and it has been suggested that toxoplasma has been evolved from a coccidian parasite pathogenic to cats. The epithelial cells of the small intestine are first invaded and the parasite multiplies in them by schizogony. When the cell is ruptured, merozoites are released. The merozoites either parasitize further intestinal cells or develop into trophozoites, which then invade the tissues in the same way that they do in other animals. Those parasites, which invade further intestinal cells either develop further schizonts or become micro- and macro-gametes. After fertilization, oocysts are formed which are shed into the lumen of the bowel and pass out with the faeces Within 48-72 hours of being voided, the oocysts form two sporocysts each containing four sporozoites. The sporozoites are infectious for all warm-blooded animals, including man. Excretion of oocysts has been found in no animals other than Felidae, and then only in two genera, *Lynx* and *Felis*, including the European Lynx, Domestic Cat, Bengal Cat, Ocelot and Jaguar. Infection occurs by ingestion of sporozoites. The oocysts containing the sporozoites are spread in dust contaminated by cat's faeces, by earthworms, cockroaches and flies. There is some mystery as to how herbivores, such as sheep, become so generally infected. It is hard to believe that pastures become widely infected with cat's faeces and it has been doubted whether infection can be spread by ingestion of infected material. The question is of importance, because one route by which man becomes infected is by eating infected meat.

It may well be that toxoplasmosis is responsible for more social problems than is generally supposed. Amongst northern races, in particular, one of the great problems of the day is that of the backward or delinquent child. Many reasons are suggested for a child's failure to progress or to conform to the rules of the community, inherited stupidity, poor social background, problems of puberty, failure to integrate with other children. However, other causes are also being sought such as low grade lead or mercury intoxication, or else some chronic infectious condition. Of the latter, toxoplasmosis is perhaps the most probable, though chronic malaria could have the same effect in children who have in the past suffered from it. It could well be that more thorough medical screening of children with problems could diminish the numbers of Borstal inmates. Any such problems are likely to be intensified at puberty; toxoplasmosis is easily diagnosed serologically and treatment is effective. The involvement of cats in the disease cycle was only discovered as recently as 1970 and must arouse the speculation that many more children are affected than was previously supposed.

In the next chapter, we shall study the next great group of pathogens which assail the human race in relation to the animal transmission of disease, namely the helminths. They too have produced pathogens, which have profoundly affected human development and history.

CHAPTER 10

Zoonoses Caused by Helminths

Introduction

We are now to consider the last great group of pathogens, which can be said to have had a serious or global effect on human ecology, namely the helminth parasites. It may be said that there are other pathogens of man especially arthropods, which are of importance, some of them zoonoses, such as the lung and mange mites, to name but two. They are competently covered by other works, such as van der Hoeden's (1964) "Zoonoses", Bisseru's (1967) "Diseases of man acquired from his pets", and Soulsby's (1974) "Parasitic Zoonoses", works which have been of value for reference in compiling this book. While noting that they exist, we need not pay them further attention.

Host-Parasite Relationships

All vertebrates have their own characteristic helminth fauna, whether they be fish, toads, snakes, birds, or mammals. Under natural conditions in the wild, few, if any, animals are not host to one or more helminths, which are either permanent residents, as with intestinal worms, or temporary or seasonal visitors as with migrating worm larvae or lungworms. Under normal circumstances, host and parasite have become adapted to each other over thousands of generations of association, and the numbers of guests are regulated by controlling mechanisms to a tolerable level. In weak or sickly animals, the worm burden may become increased above the tolerable threshold, and it is such animals that fall prey to predators; in this way the predators remove the weakest from the herd, contributing in a somewhat drastic fashion to the vigour and well-being of the species as a whole. Under conditions of domestic husbandry, in which stock are kept on pastures in high concentration, the worm burden can easily rise to harmful proportions in quite a short time; the pastures become heavily contaminated, and the animals are continually reinfecting themselves. As with other animals, man too has his natural helminth parasites, and most children at some time carry pin-worms or thread-worms, which have no adverse effect on them though their mothers would no doubt be shocked to know that they had them. In advanced countries, strict measures of hygiene and inspection of meat ensure that infection with ascarids or tapeworms are rarities; in more primitive communities, both are common. Man's tapeworms, though of no great economic significance, have a special ecological significance, since they are entirely specific to man, and both species, *Taenia saginata* and *T. solium*, are derived from his domestic animals. The larval form of *T. saginata*, known as *Cysticercus bovis*, is acquired from eating beef, and that of *T. solium*, *C. cellulosae*, from eating pork. This relationship must have become intensified since man domesticated these animals. Certainly in earlier times, when man was nomadic and his prey animals roamed over vast open spaces, conditions for any considerable build-up of these parasites did not exist; indeed, wild cattle and pigs were not his main prey animals.

There are a great many helminths, which are important zoonoses and which must be mentioned at the risk of giving a somewhat "catalogue" effect in their description. In accordance with our theme, we shall give a more detailed account of four which are of especial significance to the health of some large sections of the human race, and then deal more summarily with the remainder. The four to be specially considered are: — (i) The schistosomes (bilharzia); (ii) The filariae; (iii) trichinella; and (iv) hydatid.

Schistosomiasis

There are three species of schistosomes of especial importance in human medicine: — *Schistosoma haematobium, S. mansoni* and *S. japonicum*. They are primarily human pathogens, which occasionally infect animals, though *S. japonicum* has a wider host range. Conversely, certain other schistosomes are primarily animal parasites, which occasionally infect man. The haematobium group, thus, includes *S. intercalatum*, a parasite of cattle and antelopes in Kinshasa and West Africa, *S. bovis* and *S. matthei*, parasites of cattle, sheep and goats. The mansoni group includes *S. rodhaini* and *S. rodentarum*, parasites of rodents. *S. japonicum* can also infect cattle, sheep, goats, pigs, horses, deer, dogs, cats, weasels, shrews, moles, rats and field mice. It is highly probable that, in remote times, animals were more important as reservoirs of schistosomes, and that the human schistosomes have been evolved from those of animals as "remote" zoonoses, when water for irrigation and paddy fields became important in agriculture. According to World Health Organization statistics, in Africa and the Middle East, about 26 million of a population of 107 million suffer from schistosome infection. In China, over 100 million people, and in some areas 90% of the cattle, are infected. In the whole world, more than 200 million people suffer from the disease.

In Africa, both *S. haematobium* and *S. mansoni* are found; *S. mansoni* alone is found in Central and South America. *S. japonicum* is found in countries of East and South-east Asia, there being four geographical strains, the Chinese, the Japanese, the Philippine and the Formosan. Man is the principal host of the Philippine strain; man and animals equally of the Chinese and Japanese strains; while the Formosan strain infects chiefly animals and only exceptionally man, in whom it rarely produces eggs. This is an interesting gradation in the adaptation of a new parasite to man.

The life history of the schistosomes is all important to their distribution and control. All require freshwater snails as intermediate hosts; the snails become infected from human or animal excreta, urine or faeces, voided into the water. Schistosomes belong to the Order Trematoda and possess a marked sexual dimorphism. The females are rounded and live in a state of permanent copulation in the so-called "gynaecophoric groove" of the flattened males. The paired adults of *S. haematobium* live mainly in the veins of the urino-genital system, they produce eggs with sharp terminal spines and these eggs are passed in the urine. *S. mansoni* adults live in the inferior mesenteric veins and pass lateral-spined ova in the faeces. *S. japonicum* adult worms live mainly in the superior mesenteric veins, and ova, with much smaller terminal spines, are passed in the faeces. Each ovum releases into the water a single actively swimming "miracidium", which seeks a snail of the appropriate species. The miracidium is ingested by the snail and develops into a sporocyst, from which daughter sporocyts are produced. The sporocysts develop further and release numerous fork-tailed cercariae, which leave the snail and swim actively in the water until a suitable mammalian host is found. Entry to the host is made by penetration of the skin. The parasites then migrate by way of the blood vessels, first to the lungs, and thence to the liver. They remain in the hepatic veins for some eight weeks, during which they develop into adult males and females. After mating, they migrate in pairs to their final location. The worms are long lived, surviving in the host for as long as thirty years.

The presence of a few worms causes little systemic upset. Where the infection is heavy, serious symptoms result, which in time lead to the death of the host. In endemic areas, the most severe symptoms are seen in young people; by the time of adult life, immune mechanisms control the numbers of parasites harboured. Nevertheless, schisto-somiasis is a serious and debilitating disease with consequences often remote from the sites where the parasites are lodged. There are four stages of the syndrome. Penetration of the skin by the cercariae sets up an irritating macular or papular eruption, which may last some days; this is known as "cercarial dermatitis" or "swimmer's itch". Secondly, during their passage through the lungs, the cercariae produce trau-matic, haemorrhagic lesions with irritant cough, blood-stained saliva and patchy pneumonia; this is accompanied by irregular fever, malaise, anorexia, generalized pains, diarrhoea and eosinophilia. Thirdly, as the cercariae enter the hepatic veins, the liver becomes enlarged and tender. The phase lasts some six to eight weeks, while the cercariae develop into adults causing toxaemic and allergic symptoms, such as irregular high temperatures, urticaria, oedema of various parts of the body and eosinophilia. The fourth stage starts, when the adult worms take up position in the veins of the intestine or urinary system and begin to lay eggs. With *S. haematobium*, blood is passed in the urine; with *S. mansoni* and *S. japonicum* the faeces become dysenteric and are stained with blood. The blood comes from the points where the spiked eggs have penetrated the mucosa of the bladder or bowel. Provided the numbers of worms are small, symptoms in this phase are not severe, but they can be acute and dangerous if there are many worms present. In time, a number of ova fail to penetrate the wall of the bladder or bowel, and become stranded in the tissues or swept away in the blood stream to other sites. These ova become encapsulated and pseudotubercles are formed. Those swept away are filtered out by the liver, but some escape and pass to other organs, such as the lungs, brain, or kidneys. Those that are lodged in the brain frequently cause epileptiform symptoms. In the liver pseudotubercles are formed, and there are areas of necrosis. In chronic cases, the increasing irritation and damage to the liver leads to the formation of dense connective tissue around the tubercles, resulting in a form of cirrhosis, portal hypertension and enlargement of the spleen. Carcinoma of the liver develops in some patients. Schistosomal granulomata may also be found in the spinal cord, brain, genitalia and other organs. Sequelae distant from the site of the worms are most severe with *S. japonicum*, probably because the ova have a smaller spine and are more easily transported by the blood; they are least pronounced with *S. haema-tobium*. In chronic, endemic areas, affected persons continue for many years with their daily tasks, provided they are not over-exerted. Those, who are heavily infected become progressively more ill, and in the end die of the disease.

The schistosomiases, as diseases, are associated with water, the presence of suitable vector snails, and habits of urinating or defaecating into water where the snails are to be found. They are associated to the greatest extent with agricultural activities, especially with irrigation. Today, the disease is increasing in extent, especially in Egypt, where newer irrigation projects have increased enormously the amount of land cultivated. It is difficult to assess the overall effects of endemic schistosomiasis on a population, but it is the opinion of most experts that, where the infection rate is high, the population is severely debilitated and incapable of sustained effort and performance. Ova of *S. haematobium* have been found in the bladders of Egyptian mummies, which suggests that the infection was well established by early dynastic times. It has been suggested that the early vigour of the Egyptian people was impaired by schistosomiasis and that the decline of Egypt's importance was due, more than anything else, to its effects. We can certainly ascribe global importance to schistosome infections. Clearly it can not have been of such importance before the introduction of river based agricultural systems and one can, with reasonable certainty, attribute the appearance of the predominantly human parasites to an adaptation of those of animal origin. Thus, even though animals today play a secondary part, these diseases are "remote zoonoses". *S. haematobium* can infect wild rodents; *S. mansoni* also infects wild rodents, including gerbils and shrews. In East Africa, monkeys, particularly baboons, which use waterholes frequented by man, have been found infected with both *S. haematobium* and *S. mansoni.* Sea lions in the Cairo zoo have also been found very susceptible to both. *S. japonicum*, as already seen, infects a wide variety of domestic and wild animals; it is believed that in some parts the water buffalo, the commonest of the domestic animals in the Far East, may be the reservoir.

Filariasis (*vide* Fiennes, 1967; Orihel and Seibold, 1972)

The Filariae, or blood worms, are a group of Nematoda. The adult worms live in various sites in the body, such as the lymphatic vessels, the liver, the peritoneal cavity, or tendon sheaths. The larvae, or microfilariae, may be found in blood smears or skin scrapings. Their appearance in the blood is, in some species, diurnal and correlated with the periods of biting activity of the arthropod intermediate hosts; when not active in the blood stream, they rest in the capillaries of the lungs. Filaria are globally distributed in tropical regions, and are very common in snakes and birds, as well as in mammals. In man, they are associated with two serious diseases, "elephantiasis" and "river blindness". The reservoir hosts, apart from man himself, are other primates, though no cases of elephantiasis have been recorded in monkeys.

In monkeys, Filaria are often present in large numbers, though only one or two adults may be found. The incidence is highest in South

American monkeys, in which the infecting Filaria belong to the genera, *Dipetalonema* and *Tetrapetalonema*. These worms are occasionally found in man, but have no particular significance. The African genus, *Loa*, on the other hand, is commonly found in man and causes lesions of the eyes and skin. The worm *Loa loa* is distributed throughout the rain forest areas of Africa. The skin lesions are transient, causing oedematous swellings and itching; they may be found in many parts of the body and are recurrent. Worms traversing the eye cause irritation, congestion, lacrimation, photophobia and sometimes pain. Very occasionally, the worms enter the heart or brain, causing cardiac or cerebral symptoms. Normally, the worms live in the subcutaneous tissues and move around fairly rapidly. As many as 40 adult worms have been found in one person. *Loa spp* are transmitted by tabanid biting flies, *Chrysops langi*. These flies bite at all canopy levels in the forests and are attracted to the smell of wood fires, thus locating human victims. Various species of *Loa* occur in forest primates; those of baboons and gorillas are the same as those found in man.

Elephantiasis in man is caused by species of *Brugia*, *B. bancrofti* in Africa and *B. malayi* in the Far East. Persons of all ages are commonly infected with these worms. Patients suffer from intermittent fever and swelling of the limbs with lymphangitis and lymphadenitis. Elephantiasis of the legs or scrotum, with hydrocele, orchitis, and epididymitis, frequently follow, but is commoner in the African form of the disease. These symptoms are due to the presence of adult worms in lymphatic vessels. Brugia are transmitted by mosquitos, and are found in monkeys, as well as cats and dogs and some wild species, such as tiger, moon rat and pangolin. In infected areas, 10-20% of the population may be infected.

The filarial worm, *Onchocerca volvulus*, is commonly found in areas of East and West Africa, and in Central America, where there are fast-flowing streams. The adults are found in the skin of man, where they are associated with unpleasant and characteristic lesions, onchocercal dermatitis. The microfilariae, during their migrations, frequently find their way to the eyes, causing keratitis and iritis; the results are impaired vision and frequently blindness (River Blindness). Eye lesions appear to be more frequent in West Africa than East, a high proportion of the population becoming blind in some parts. Onchocerca are transmitted by blackflies, *Simulium damnosum*. These flies breed only in fast-running streams, laying their eggs on freshwater crustacea on which the larvae develop. *O. volvulus* were thought formerly to be solely parasites of man, but it has been found that in some parts of West Africa gorillas are extensively infected, and it is possible that chimpanzees may be infected also.

Apart from the specific lesions mentioned, filarial infections cause eosinophilia and chronic anaemia, and are responsible for a great deal of ill health and suffering in most parts of the tropics. Animal reservoirs are probably not of great importance in maintaining infection; yet they exist and attempts to eliminate these diseases from man could well be frustrated by reintroduction from animal sources. River Blindness is fortunately limited in its distribution, because of the breeding requirements of the infected flies. Elephantiasis, on the other hand, is widespread in Asia and Africa, causing great disability and distress in a large number of persons.

Trichinelliasis

Trichinelliasis is caused by a minute nematode, *Trichinella spiralis*, the females being up to 4 mm and the males 2 mm in length. These worms, however, cause one of the most serious of the helminthiases, the life of the host being often in danger from the infection. Epidemics have been common from the Middle Ages, if not earlier, though the cause of the trouble was not formerly understood. The adult worms live in the lower part of the small intestine and the upper parts of the large bowel, where they do little harm. The parasite, however, has a unique life cycle, and it is on this that the serious symptoms depend. Infection is by the ingestion of meat containing viable larvae. Even cooked meat is dangerous, since cooking temperatures are often insufficient to kill the larvae, especially in such products as meat pies and sausages. The larvae develop directly into adults in the intestines in less than two days. Copulation then takes place between the sexes and live larvae are produced by the female; the larvae escape through the vulva into the lumen of the intestine, being shed for several weeks until the female dies. For further development, the larvae must be laid in the villi of the small intestine; they then invade the central lacteals and are carried by the lymph through the mesenteric glands to the thoracic duct and thence to the vena cava, heart, lungs and arterial circulation. The larvae are so small, that they can easily travel through the capillaries, yet they cause extensive haemorrhages and pneumonic lesions in the lungs. The larvae penetrate the tissues, and those that enter skeletal muscles develop further. They penetrate the muscle sheaths and appear within 6-7 days inside the muscle fibre itself. The muscle fibre degenerates and the larva rolls itself into the characteristic spiral and becomes encapsulated. Although encapsulated, the larva is not inactive; it absorbs food and oxygen, derived from the detritus of cell destruction, and from the capillaries which are formed round the capsule. In infected animals, hundreds, even thousands, of larvae are found in every gramme of muscle tissue.

Trichinella can infect almost every form of mammalian host, which consumes flesh, both carnivore and omnivore; obviously herbivores will not normally acquire infection. Its incidence is highest in Arctic lands, such as Alaska and Northern Canada, where large numbers of predators feed on a comparatively small number of primary producers, and also on each other. Foxes eat rodents and weasels; bears and wolves eat foxes and so a chain of infection is established. Infection can also be acquired by eating wolves, walrus, seal, bears and husky dogs, all possible items of diet in an Eskimo menu. Infection of man in arctic regions may be as high as 90%. The Arctic apart, the source of infection in man is usually the pig or pig products. As an omnivore, the pig will eat wild rodents and rats are regarded as the primary wild reservoir. It has often been surmised that religious bans on the consumption of pork, as with Moslems and Jews, stem from the fear of illness associated with it, though the cause was not understood. Apart from the Arctic regions, trichinelliasis was widespread in northern Europe, in north and south America, and in those Asian countries, where pork was eaten. It is absent from tropical countries, including the whole of Africa and the Pacific Islands, and from Australia.

Heavy infections of trichinelliasis produce severe clinical symptoms, of which two are characteristic, namely high eosinophil counts in the blood and oedema of the face below the orbits. The temperature is irregular; there is general malaise; pains in the muscles and joints, and coughing. The condition is sometimes confused with Rheumatic Fever. The most severe symptoms appear in the early invasive stage of infection. Pain is severe in the muscles of the extremities and chest, and in the eyeballs. Breathing becomes difficult and a painful cough develops. There are sometimes haemorrhages in the retina and cerebral symptoms may appear. The patient then, either dies in coma from cardiac or respiratory failure; or, symptoms regress, though survivors often become chronic invalids. The mortality in trichinelliasis varies according to the intensity of the infection; in severe epidemics, it may be as high as 16%. The larval worms may be found in any muscles of the body, but especially in the muscles of respiration, intercostals and diaphragm.

The high incidence of trichinelliasis in Arctic regions is of some interest. Palaeolithic man, living under ice age conditions, could well have been quite heavily infected with this parasite. His normal diet was acquired from reindeer and other herbivores, but he must surely have supplemented this with rodents, bears, foxes, or wolves, when he could acquire them. This position is in contrast with other diseases that we have considered, most of which are "new diseases" associated with a changed way of life. The rat ⟶ pig ⟶ man cycle developed in more southerly countries could well qualify as a new form of the disease, associated with domestication or semi-domestication of pigs.

Hydatidosis

Hydatid disease presents some similar features. The minute adult tapeworms, *Echinococcus granulosus*, are parasites of canine predators, including wolf and jackal. The intermediate hosts are their prey animals, including reindeer, caribou, cattle, sheep, goats, pigs, horses and zebras. Man is normally a dead-end host, who becomes accidentally infected if his food becomes contaminated with canine faeces. In Artic regions, where wolves prey on caribou or reindeer, there is a simple cycle of infection from wolf to reindeer and reindeer to wolf. The reindeer acquire infection from ground contaminated with wolves' faeces, and the wolves contract infection from eating the viscera of the reindeer; the reindeer become so incapacitated by the infection that they fall easy prey to the wolves.

It is characteristic of tapeworms that the larval worms usually cause more serious diseases than the adults. There are three groups of tapeworms, which produce different forms of larvae: —

Adult	Larval form
Taenia	*Cysticerus*
Multiceps	*Coenurus*
Echinococcus	Hydatid

The first two genera are similar, except in the larval form in which the *Multiceps* larva produces many heads (*Coenurus*), whereas the *Taenia* larva produces only a single head. In the hydatid cyst, on the other hand, new larval heads continually bud from a germinal layer of the cyst. Because of this, the hydatid cyst will grow continuously in a parasitized organ, until it may eventually be destroyed and the host animal dies. The organ most frequently affected by hydatid is the right lobe of the liver, but lungs, kidneys, bones and brain may also be affected. Sometimes, the cyst will burst and metastatic cysts become developed. Infection with a single cyst is often not particularly serious; indeed, the host may remain symptomless for years and the cyst may die, shrink and become calcified. The severity of symptoms depends mainly on the organ affected, the results being due mainly to pressure effects. However, in extreme cases the patient may be affected with many cysts, even hundreds, which expand the abdomen to large proportions and cause considerable destruction of the affected organs. The presence of cysts in brain, kidney, heart and spinal cord are particularly serious. When a cyst ruptures, embolism of various organs may occur, especially of the lungs.

Multiple hydatidosis usually occurs under rather special conditions; in these circumstances, the disease has become a major scourge. In Wales and Australia, and other countries too, the incidence of hydatid has been very high amongst sheep-shearers. The sheep are rounded up, and corralled for shearing. Sick or thrifty sheep are killed and the carcases are thrown to the sheepdogs, who consume the viscera including any cysts. The corrals are heavily contaminated with the dogs' droppings, and the shearers can hardly avoid getting their hands contaminated, and so becoming infected when they eat. The distribution of hydatid is worldwide, but the main endemic areas are where the sheep ⟶ dog ⟶ man cycle can be maintained, such as the southern regions of south America, South Africa, southern Australia, New Zealand, Mediterranean countries, northern Europe and the more northerly parts of North America. The disease was formerly very prevalent in Iceland, but has been controlled by preventing sheepdogs from having access to sheep entrails.

Other Nematodes

Of the other nematodes, which have some importance to man as a zoonosis, we may mention the Guinea Worm, *Dracunculus medinensis.* This worm is common in the drier parts of the tropics, Arabia, southern Asia, and West and Central Africa. It is also present in China, Korea, Indonesia, Fiji and the West Indies. Reservoir hosts are dog, cat, fox, raccoon, mink, horses, cattle and monkeys. However, infection usually passes from man to man through the intermediate host, which is a freshwater crustacean, *Cyclops.* Man is infected by drinking water containing these creatures. The worm larvae are released in the stomach and penetrate its wall, developing into adults in about a year. The adult worms are long and narrow, and they move slowly and continuously in a tortuous fashion through the connective tissues. The males copulate early on and the females, when filled with larvae, move towards the surface of the body. A blister is formed beneath the skin, which eventually bursts and the anterior end of the female protrudes to the outside. The cuticle is removed from the head of the worm by the body reactions, and permits the uterus to come to the surface and release the larvae, which emerge in a drop of whitish fluid when contact is made with fresh water. Hundreds of larvae emerge, which seek another *Cyclops.* Eventually the entire worm leaves the wound and healing takes place. The process of removing the worm is often hastened by rolling it slowly day by day over a match stick. There are no serious effects from Guinea Worm.

Another nematode with an unusual life history is *Strongyloides.* These parasites are common in tropical and sub-tropical countries, and are found also in dogs, cats and monkeys. Infection in man can be serious and deaths have occurred from it. The serious nature is the result of the life history. There are at least three species of *Strongyloides,* *S. cebus* and *S. fulleborni* from New and Old World monkeys, and *S. stercoralis,* which infects man and is probably the same as that which infects dogs and cats. Whether the monkey species can infect man is not known, but they probably can do so. *Strongyloides* are small worms, having alternate free-living and parasitic generations. The adults are found in the large bowel, in which they cause ulceration and sometimes perforation. The fertilised eggs produce rhabditoid larvae in the bowel, which pass to the exterior; they feed and grow in the free state, until they metamorphose into long filariform larvae. These larvae penetrate the skin of a new host. They enter the blood stream, and pass to the heart and lungs; they break out into the lung alveoli and there develop further. They then pass up the respiratory tract and are swallowed to start a new generation in the large intestine. The female becomes fertilised during the migration and, on reaching the intestine, she burrows into the mucosa and lays her eggs. The dangers from these worms occur when some worms develop directly into filariform larvae in the intestine and the free-living stage is by-passed; these filariform larvae reinfect the same host and, in this way, a very heavy infection can be built up from an initially low level. The damage caused by the burrowing of the female into the bowel mucosa can be serious; the lesions sometimes become infected and pyaemia or septicaemia can result with fatal consequences.

Larva Migrans

The wandering habits of many nematode larvae cause varying forms of disease from the mildly irritating to those that are serious. These are known as *larva migrans* and two forms are recognised: — 1. Cutaneous Larva Migrans, which is the cutaneous form also called "creeping eruption". This is usually associated with penetration of the skin by hookworm larvae, but other worms such as *Strongyloides*, *Gnathostoma*, and larvae of the cattle hookworm, *Bunostomum*, may also be responsible. In an abnormal host, the infection is likely to prove abortive, so that creeping eruption can be caused by worm larvae of non-pathogenic species. We are here concerned with: — 2. Visceral Larva Migrans, and especially with that form associated with the roundworms of the dog and cat, *Toxocara canis* and *T. cati*, which can have serious consequences for children. The life history of *Toxocara* in dogs is unusual. Almost all puppies are infected pre-natally by the bitch with second stage larvae. They mature in about 21 days in the puppies' intestines; the faeces may contain up to 15 000 eggs per gramme. The suckling bitch eats the faeces of the puppies and reinfects herself thereby with first stage larvae; they become second stage larvae and become encysted in the lungs and somatic tissues. This is a most unusual feature of the life history, which does not occur with *Toxocara cati*. When pregnancy occurs, these larvae are mobilised and pass to the uterus and so infect the new generation of puppies before birth; in the puppies, they pass by way of the liver and lungs to the stomach. It is only the puppies, which pass infective ova for some 8-10 weeks. It is the ova in the faeces of puppies, by which children become infected, but infection can also pass to mice, guinea pigs, other rodents, rabbits and birds. Dogs may, also, become infected by eating an infected rodent, so that even if dogs were cleared of *Toxocara* a reservoir exists in nature by which infection could be re-established. *Toxocara cati* has a straightforward life history, in which the adult males and females live in the gut of the host at all ages. Cats can acquire infection from each other, or, as with the dog worm, from eating an infected mouse. Both *T. canis* and *T. cati* are worldwide in distribution. *T. canis* can infect virtually all Canidae, including domestic dogs, foxes, wolves, jackals, dingos, hyaenas and raccoons among the Procyonidae. *T. cati* infects a great many of the Felidae, including the domestic cat, wild cat, leopard, cheetah, puma, tiger, lion, jaguar, serval, lynx, bobcat and rarely foxes.

Visceral Larva Migrans causes a syndrome, which may be serious in children. Internal organs, such as the liver, lungs, eyes, brain, heart, kidneys and lymphatic glands may be invaded and suffer from granulomata with serious tissue damage. The syndrome is accompanied by serious intermittent fever, loss of appetite, cough, asthmatic episodes, together with abdominal discomfort, muscular aches and pains, and neurological symptoms. Invasion of children's eyes by *Toxocara* larvae is particularly serious. The affected eye becomes enlarged and granulomata of the retina are caused. In many cases, the affected eye has had to be removed, the parasite being lodged near the macula and optic disc.

The hookworms are of no importance as zoonoses, except in so far as alien hookworms can cause the symptoms of Cutaneous Larva Migrans. Bowel infections in man are only caused by specifically human species of *Ancylostoma* and *Necator*.

Other Trematodes

Amongst the trematodes, the common "liver fluke" of cattle and sheep, *Fasciola hepatica*, is occasionally found in the human liver. In addition to cattle and sheep, this fluke can infect a number of other hosts, including goats, pigs, horses, donkeys, camels, llamas, vicunas, deer, antelopes, elephants, rabbits, hares, coypus, squirrels, kangaroos, beavers, dogs, monkeys, rats and mice. Rabbits and coypus are the most important wild hosts in most parts of the world, including Britain. In tropical regions, an allied form, *Fasciola magna*, is found, and this too occasionally infects man. Like the schistosomes, liver flukes are transmitted through a secondary host, which is a snail. The infective metacercariae crawl on to the leaves of green herbage and are ingested when this is eaten. In Britain, most cases have arisen from contaminated watercress.

Another fluke, which commonly infects man, is *Fasciolopsis buski.* This very large fluke inhabits the small intestine of man and the main reservoir host is the pig; occasionally dogs are infected also. Millions of persons are infected in China, Formosa, Vietnam, Thailand, Bengal and Assam in India, and parts of Indonesia. The infective metacercariae encyst on freshwater plants, such as water caltrop, water chestnuts, and water bamboo. The worms cause deep ulceration of the intestinal mucosa, causing severe abdominal pain simulating peptic ulcer. If infection is heavy, the lumen of the intestine may be blocked, leading to ascites and sudden death.

Clonorchis sinensis is a trematode, which inhabits the bile ducts in the liver and, rarely, the pancreatic ducts, of man, dogs, cats, rats, pigs, weasels, mink, badgers and other fish-eating carnivores throughout the Far East. Four and a half million people are said to be infected in Japan and Korea alone. The results of a heavy infection can be serious with hepatitis, cholangitis, cirrhosis, biliary obstruction and stone formation. The cercariae pass from a snail host into a fish, where metacercariae become encysted in the muscles.

Rather similar trematodes are *Opisthorchis felineus* and *O. viverrini.* The main host of *O. felineus* is the cat, but man, dog, fox and wild fish-eating carnivores are infected in various European countries. The trematodes reside in the bile ducts, causing hepatitis and cirrhosis. *O. vivverrini* is endemic in Thailand, where a large part of the population is infected as a result of eating raw fish with rice. The reservoir animals are domestic dogs, cats and, in the wild, the civet cat (*Felis vivverrina*) and other fish-eating carnivores. The flukes live in the bile ducts and cause cirrhosis and carcinoma.

Paragonimus westermanni is another trematode of man which is found in the Far East, parts of south-east Asia and Nigeria. The flukes are parasites of dogs, cats and wild carnivores, like the fox, leopard, tiger, mink and civet cat. The infective stage is found in crabs and crayfish, in which the metacercariae are present in muscle, gills and other organs. In man, the larval metacercariae penetrate the wall of the duodenum, and migrate across the peritoneal cavity to enter the lungs through the diaphragm. The adult parasites live for years in cyst-like cavities in the lungs. However, some flukes lose their way in the peritoneal cavity and become lodged in other organs than the lungs, such as the liver, gut wall, mesenteric lymph nodes, muscles, testes and brain. Pneumothorax is common during the course of infection, and secondary pyogenic organisms may cause lung abscesses. The disease is often complicated by tuberculosis.

Other Cestodes

Amongst the Cestodes, the taenias and cysticercoses have already been mentioned. The taenias are not parasites of any other primate than man, their life history being associated with a carnivorous diet. Other members of the taenia group occur only in carnivores, and all have a larval stage, the cysticercus, which is to be found in prey animals. The common tapeworms of other primates belong to the genus *Bertiella* of which there are seven species. They are transmitted by ingestion of the secondary host, which is believed to be a free-living mite. Three of these species have been found in man, *B. mucronata*, a parasite of vervet monkeys and chimpanzees, *B. satyri*, a parasite of orang-utans and gibbons, and *B. studeri*, which can infect chimpanzees, orang-utans, gibbons, baboons, macaques and some cercopitheque monkeys. Dogs can also be infected with these worms; in man infection is confined to children. Children can also be infected with a dog tapeworm, *Dipylidium caninum*, which belongs like *Bertiella* to the Order Anoplocephalidae. This is transmitted both to dogs and to children by dog fleas, which are the intermediate hosts.

The largest tapeworm of man, indeed known in nature, is *Diphyllobothrium latum*, also known as the fish tapeworm. It lives in the small intestine of man, other normal hosts being dog, cat, bear, fox, mongoose, walrus, sea lion, mink, leopard and pig. Dogs are very important in spreading infection. Operculated eggs are passed in thousands in the faeces of an infected animal. They hatch in fresh water and the ciliated embryos swim actively until swallowed by freshwater Crustacea, *Cyclops*, in which they develop into nine-hooked "procercoids", the first larval stage. The procercoids are eaten by fish, such as perch, salmon, trout, barbel, pike, or sometimes frogs. In these secondary hosts, the procercoids develop into second stage larvae, known as plerocercoids, which become encysted in the muscles or the roe. The adult develops in the final host when the fish is eaten. Distribution of this tapeworm is worldwide, but is highest where sanitary conditions are poor and fish are eaten raw or partially cooked. The worm causes anaemia and interferes with the absorption of Vitamin B_{12} from the bowel.

In addition to the adult tapeworms, to which man is sometimes host, he can also harbour the larval stages of some of these parasites. He sometimes even harbours the larval stages of his own tapeworms, *Cysticerous bovis* and *C. cellulosae*, normally found in beef and pork. He may become infected in two ways, either by eating food contaminated with infected faeces, possibly his own, or by auto-infection within the intestine. *C. bovis* is rare, but *C. cellulosae* not uncommon. The infection is usually confined to the skeletal muscles, but can be serious in the rare cases when the eyes or central nervous system are involved. It was reported in 1933, that an average of 97 soldiers had been invalided yearly from the British army during a period of five years because of epilepsy caused by cysticerci.

Coenurus larvae have been recorded in man from four species of the tapeworm *Multiceps*, the adults of which infect Canidae, such as dogs and jackals. *Coenurus* cysts normally occur in sheep and rabbits, and man is an accidental host. *Coenurus cerebralis*, the larva of *Multiceps multiceps*, is the most dangerous, because it has a special affinity for the brain and spinal cord. It is the cause of "staggers" or "gid" in sheep, and has been found also in wild goats and sheep, and in gazelles. Infection in man can be serious, the symptoms resembling those of a brain tumour. The larvae of *M. serialis*, known as *Coenurus serialis*, are normally found in rabbits, but also in squirrels, coypu, monkeys and other animals. In man, usually young children, the coenuri are found mainly beneath the skin. They have been found in all continents, except Australia. Dogs are the main source of infection. The third species of *Coenurus* that has been found in man is *C. glomeratus*, which normally occurs in the form of small cysts in the internal organs of small rodents in some parts of Africa. Three cases have been recorded in man. The host of the adult worm is unknown.

Finally, the larva of a tapeworm allied to *Diphyllobothrium latum*, *D. mansoni*, occasionally occurs in man. These are known as *Sparganum* (*S. mansoni*), and the disease as sparganosis. The adult worms are found in dogs, cats and other carnivores, and are acquired by eating the intermediate hosts, frogs, lizards, snakes and birds harbouring the plerocercoid stage. The infection is prevalent in Korea, where raw snake flesh is eaten for medicinal purposes; otherwise infections with the adult worms are not found in man. Infection with the spargana or larvae occurs in Indonesia, Africa, the United States and to the greatest extent in China. It is probably acquired from drinking water containing water fleas. In the Far East, infection also occurs from the habit of applying raw frog's flesh to sore eyes, when the plerocercoids transfer themselves to the eyes attracted by the warmth; blindness may result.

With this account, we end our review of helminths as zoonoses. Worms and their hosts have been inseparable companions over many millions of years, and man has been no exception to the rule.

Nevertheless, his odd habits and ways of life have exposed him to certain hazards, which were unimportant to the nomadic creature of earlier times. Much of the trouble rests with unhygienic habits, which, having persisted from the earliest days of civilization, are extraordinarily difficult to reform. To conquer bilharzia, for example, it is only necessary to refrain from voiding excreta into fresh water, where there are snails. In spite of intensive propaganda, these habits continue.

PART III
Man-Animal Relationships in the Spread of Morbid Conditions

CHAPTER 11

Man and his Animals

Introduction

It is an ecological fact of life that man has lived in association with animals he has domesticated for a very long time. He had domesticated dogs long before the days of agriculture, and by early Neolithic times there had appeared small breeds of pet dogs which were presumably kept in the home in close contact with both adults and children. In dynastic Egyptian times, cats were being kept and one recalls the charming domestic scenes in the tombs of the nobles, where husband and wife are portrayed eating their breakfast with the cat eating a fish under the table. It is another ecological fact of life that neither dogs nor cats can be deterred from hunting and consuming small animals, such as rats and mice, from which they can acquire organisms and infections harmful to human beings. With the agricultural revolution, farm animals also came to be domesticated, horses, cattle, sheep, goats, pigs and poultry amongst others. Until recent times, farm animals were often kept in crowded, insanitary conditions, which favoured the spread of diseases, some of them harmful to man.

Some dangers from farm animals, such as tuberculosis and brucellosis, have given concern for a long time, and drastic measures for their control or elimination have greatly reduced the risks. Strangely, it is only during the past twenty years or so that realisation has dawned that pet animals, such as dogs, cats, cage birds and even tortoises, can also carry diseases, which can be potentially dangerous especially to children. The subject is emotive and many people would rather that these dangers had remained undiscovered. Accidents and tragedies are few and nobody suggests that, because of them, the age old practice of keeping pets could or should be abandoned. To do so would be socially undesirable; to many families, a home is not a home without some kind of pet and many think that association with pets provides a beneficial emotional outlet for children, which is highly desirable and outweighs the risks involved. At many schools, too, there is a pets' corner, and it is regarded as part of a child's education to handle and communicate with animals. However, parents, school teachers, education officers and the doctors who advise them, should be aware that there are risks from animals; what these risks are; and how to minimize them. With proper care and precaution, the risks become almost negligible. Anything written here is not intended to discourage the keeping of pets, except for monkeys for reasons explained below.

It is not my object here to catalogue all the diseases of domestic or captive animals, which could be transmitted to man. Such has been comprehensively achieved by Bisseru (1967) in his excellent book: "Diseases of Man acquired from his Pets." Much valuable information is also contained in the "UFAW Handbook of Laboratory Animals", of which I had the privilege of editing the latest (1976) edition. I shall attempt here to highlight the more serious dangers from pet and domestic animals and convey advice as to sensible precautions that should be taken. I shall start with Primates, which are of exceptional danger to man, both young and old, and which in my opinion should never be kept as pets where there are children in the house, and only by adults who are well aware of what they are doing.

Primates

In spite of their close phylogenetic relationships, man's disease patterns have diverged widely in almost every way from those of his cousin primates. Diseases, which man shares with apes and monkeys were reviewed at greater length in Fiennes' (1967) "Zoonoses of Primates, and a comprehensive review of simian diseases is to be found in Fiennes' (1972) "Pathology of Simian Primates" Parts I and II. Many of man's helminth parasites are those of a predator; those of other primates resemble more those of non-predators or even of prey species. The respiratory pathogens, which affect man, such as the Rhinoviruses, the Myxoviruses and the Pneumococci, are so distinct from those of other primates that they can only with difficulty be infected with them. Such differences are the result of ecological separation, which has been intensified by man's newer ways of life. However, the phylogenetic resemblances have the consequence that many simian pathogens have a greatly enhanced virulence for man. Yellow Fever and B virus (*Herpesvirus simiae*) are two instances which have already been discussed. The pathogens introduced by imported primates fall into three categories: — (i) their own natural commensals, such as B virus; (ii) pathogens acquired after capture usually from human sources and which they transmit to persons in a different continent, who are not normally affected; such are tuberculosis and infectious hepatitis; (iii) diseases hitherto unknown, which suddenly appear in persons who come into contact with the imported animals; the latest instance of this is Marburg Disease. One might add rabies to this list, to which monkeys sometimes succumb after importation; rabies is usually contracted from dogs after capture, but instances are known in which the animal was already incubating the disease at the time of capture. We shall study in greater detail the instances of shigellosis, infectious hepatitis, Marburg Disease and Rabies.

Shigellosis of Primates

Monkeys often become seriously ill or die from shigellosis. The infection is usually contracted from contact with human populations; sometimes the monkeys are endemically infected in the wild but only those that live in contact with human settlements, such as the "temple" monkeys of India; alternatively, they may become infected between capture and shipment. While many monkeys become sick and die from shigellosis, a proportion become recidivist or asymptomatic. The difficulty of detecting infection in monkeys that are asymptomatic, or even infected for that matter, has been mentioned in an earlier chapter; this means that, even when monkeys have been properly screened and quarantined, they may still be dangerous both for human beings and for other monkeys in the colony.

The most serious incident of shigellosis contracted from imported monkeys was that described by Bach *et al.* (1931). Seventeen cases of dysentery occurred following contact with a single shipment of monkeys; three persons, all children under five years old, died. *Shigella flexneri* type Y was isolated from the patients. All the monkeys had at some time suffered from diarrhoea or passed bloody stools, but had recovered before the outbreak and *faecal cultures were negative.* One monkey relapsed and died and one was sacrificed. Shigellae were isolated from both monkeys, but only from the small intestine and stomach. A further case described by Carpenter and Sandiford (1952) reveals how slight a contact with a monkey can result in severe bacillary dysentery. To quote: —

> One monkey grasped the child's ice cream cone, briefly touching the ice cream which was then licked by the child. Two days later the child was ill and refused lunch. Diarrhoea began by evening, and two days later was mucoid and bloody. Two six day courses of succinyl-suphathiazole were required to render the child's stool free from shigellae. The bacilli cultured from the stools were *Sh. flexneri* 103 Z (= 4b) . . . All the monkeys had been in the pet shop for nearly two years and free from diarrhoea the entire time. *After considerable effort, Sh. flexneri* 103 Z (= 4b) was isolated from the monkey.

(Author's italics). The child would probably have died but for treatment.

Infectious Hepatitis of Primates

Infectious hepatitis went for long unrecognised in simians. Infected animals do not show characteristic symptoms and existence of the disease was only suspected because of a higher than normal incidence in persons who came in contact with infected animals. One striking example occurred at the Holloman Air Force base in New Mexico, where a large colony of chimpanzees was maintained for space research. The incidence of infectious hepatitis amongst persons, who came in contact with newly imported chimpanzees from West Africa, was 52% as against 0·4% amongst other personnel employed there and 0·2% in Otero County, New Mexico. Infected apes and monkeys show impaired liver function, as revealed by tests of liver function. By use of such tests, a general survey of primates was made throughout the United States during 1963. Of the 78 cases investigated up to that date, chimpanzees were thought to have been the source of infection in 61, woolly monkeys (*Lagothrix spp.*) in nine, a gorilla in four and Celebes Apes (*Cynopithecus niger*) in four. Thus New and Old World species are involved in the same way.

Since these early studies, a great deal of work has been done on infectious hepatitis, which was reviewed by Smetana (1972). It is now known to be a common disease of chimpanzees but can infect a number of other species of apes and monkeys, patas, woolly monkeys, marmosets and others; baboons do not appear to contract infection. Infection is usually free from clinical symptoms, though sometimes severe illness and even death results particularly in young animals. Animals that have recovered from infection are immune to reinfection. Research into the etiology of the disease has been hampered as a result, because so many monkeys resist experimental infection presumably because they have been infected previously. Because of the absence of clinical symptoms, infection can quickly spread through a colony undetected; then all the inmates become immune and useless for research on the disease. At the same time, persons in contact with the monkeys become infected from an unsuspected source.

Infectious hepatitis was shown by Findlay *et al.* (1939) to be caused by a virus more than 30 years ago, but all attempts to find an animal model ended in failure, and no success was achieved in attempts to culture it. Eventually, Holmes *et al.* (1972) were able to infect marmosets (*Saguinus spp.*) and it became possible to study the characteristics of the virus and the ways in which it is transmitted. Infection occurs by ingestion of material contaminated with infected faeces. The virus has, however, the ability to survive for a considerable time in water, and contamination of drinking water has been the cause of some outbreaks. The virus can also survive in sea water and infection can be acquired from oysters, clams and other shellfish, when eaten.

The virus of infectious hepatitis is usually regarded as primarily human rather than simian. The high infection rate in some batches of newly imported chimpanzees and some monkeys is likely to be the result of contact with infected persons in the country of origin. Tests of liver function usually show that some are infected on arrival, others becoming infected later, until all have contracted the disease; after two to three months all have recovered and are immune. No fatal cases have so far been reported in man from simian contact. Nevertheless, the disease is serious in man, fatalities in outbreaks varying from 2% to 10%. The recovery period also is prolonged and the symptoms very unpleasant. Newly imported simians should be handled with care for this as for other reasons, and routine liver function tests are to be recommended during the acclimatisation period.

Marburg Disease

Marburg Disease provides an instance of those diseases, formerly unknown, which suddenly appear as a result of simian contacts. A review of this disease was given by Simpson (1972). There were three small episodes in the August and September of 1967 amongst laboratory workers in Germany and Yugoslavia. The disease was not again encountered, until a natural outbreak occurred in Ethiopia and Soudan in 1976; meanwhile its origins were obscure. The original outbreaks were traced to a single consignment of vervet monkeys, *Cercopithecus aethiops*, shipped from the same source in Uganda within a few days. The monkeys had been held in quarantine at London airport, where they came in contact with birds and other exotic animals. In all there were 29 human cases, of which five were secondary infections arising from contact with patients in hospital. Seven from amongst the primary cases died; all of the primary infections were derived from handling the blood or tissues from the monkeys, which were killed shortly after their arrival in the laboratories.

None of the monkeys, from which the infection was derived, showed any signs of illness. However, experimental infection of monkeys, vervet (*Cercopithecus aethiops*), rhesus (*Macaca mulatta*) and squirrel (*Saimiri sciureus*), showed that the virus was extremely virulent for monkeys and all the experimental animals died. The monkeys contracted the disease after an incubation period of two to ten days, depending on the size of the inoculum and the route of administration. They developed a mild fever at first; no overt signs of sickness were apparent until some 48 hours before death, in most cases 6-13 days after inoculation.

144 Zoonoses and the Origins and Ecology of Human Disease

It has been concluded that the monkeys involved in the outbreak had contracted the disease prior to shipment from Uganda. However, it seemed unlikely that monkeys were the primary hosts of the virus until the more recent natural outbreak, in which they were undoubtedly involved. Kalter (1972) had disagreed with this conclusion on the grounds that a number of simian species, including vervets, had been found in his laboratories to reveal antibody to the virus in blood sera. He had concluded that a focus of infection must exist in African monkeys; his views appear to have been vindicated. Virus is present in the urine and saliva of infected animals and natural infection could occur by aerosol.

Rabies in Primates

Rabies contracted from apes and monkeys has so far not been reported in human beings. In spite of this, in the United Kingdom primates have been brought under the restriction of anti-rabies legislation, so that they must be compulsorily quarantined on approved premises for at least six months after importation. Although the risk of contracting rabies from monkeys is small, this regulation is sensible, both because of the terrible results of rabies in man, and because monkeys need to be quarantined for other diseases, known and unknown, which are so dangerous. The new regulations pose problems for importers of primates and for laboratories where primates are used. They also make the animals more expensive, and they have successfully and rightly killed the trade in pet monkeys.

The numbers of imported monkeys, which are known to have contracted rabies are extremely small in relation to the numbers of imports; they have been reviewed by Fiennes (1972). However, the reported cases may well not reflect the true numbers, since infected monkeys rarely show symptoms by which rabies could be diagnosed; they invariably die, but the cause of death may well be unrecognised. Infected monkeys do not usually attack human beings unless they are teased, and in one case where the owner was bitten he did not contract rabies. It is said that in human rabies the saliva is not infected with virus, and man to man infection is unknown; whether this is true of simian primates has not been ascertained. Obviously, it would be foolish to place reliance on this possibility. The potential dangers from unrecognised rabies in monkeys are illustrated by the following case, described by Boulger (1966) as summarised by Fiennes (1972):—

> The affected animal was one of a consignment of thirty three *Macaca mulatta*, received at the Medical Research Council in Hampstead, London, England; the monkeys were collected from various sources in India and imported by air. On day forty seven, the monkey, an adult female, was noticed to be off its food and inclined to cower in the back of the cage and bite at its fingers and hands. By day

fifty one, the self inflicted wounds were so severe that the monkey had to be killed. Before death, it showed no aggressiveness nor aversion to drinking, and there was no obvious paralysis. The existence of rabies was confirmed by histological examination of cerebral tissues and injection of material into mice.

Had this monkey not been at an institute, where comprehensive tissue studies are made on all animals that die, rabies would never have been detected.

In a further case also quoted by Fiennes (1972), which occurred at the Yerkes Primate Center in Atlanta, Georgia, a monkey imported from the Philippines also died of rabies without showing diagnostic symptoms. In this case, it was calculated that the incubation period must have been *at least* five months and probably a good deal more. In a third case reported from Texas, a monkey died four to five weeks after being bitten by a rabid dog. This monkey showed no symptoms, except that it became very friendly and died suddenly.

It is evident that monkeys may not only show no symptoms indicative of rabies, but the disease could develop after their six month period of screening and quarantine. No confidence can, therefore, be felt about the safety of monkeys in respect of rabies or shigellosis even when the normal quarantine period is ended.

In studying the zoonotic relationships of man with his animals, simian primates have purposely been studied first. These animals are unfortunately essential at present to the study of many human diseases. Without the use of monkeys, vaccines could not have been developed against poliomyelitis. Without the use of monkeys, it may be impossible to discover the true causes of cancer and the means to overcome it. However, monkeys especially if newly imported should never be handled, except by properly trained and qualified staff using all possible means of protection. In view of the dangers involved, it is surprising how few disasters have occurred from buying a pet monkey for children from the local pet shop; when they have occurred, the consequences have been serious. Not only is this true of pet monkeys, as is shown by the B virus and Marburg tragedies. It is best, then, not to keep monkeys or use them in experiments unless really necessary.

Household Pets

The main pets kept in family households are dogs and cats, despite which a great many other animals are to be found in many households and also in schools. Children delight in keeping small animals, a healthy practice if well regulated and not one to be discouraged. Such animals vary from fish in aquaria, goldfish in bowls, snakes, tortoises, birds, rodents of many kinds, rabbits, hedgehogs, skunks and many others. Dogs and cats are a special case, so let us first study the dangers, if any, from keeping the more unusual pets.

Exotic Pets

Fishes in aquaria and bowls appear to represent no hazard, nor do tadpoles and frogs. Reptiles, such as snakes, lizards and tortoises, are a different matter. They carry in their guts a bacterial flora that is different from that of warm-blooded animals. Bacteria, such as *Escherichia coli*, normally resident in the gut of mammals, can prove pathogenic to them. On the other hand, they commonly harbour species of salmonella, which are commensal though pathogenic to mammals. Some of these commensals are harmless; others may be pathogenic in human patients, especially children. Tortoises, in particular, have been incriminated over causing outbreaks of salmonellosis in children. In Britain, such outbreaks have been associated with tortoises, *Testudo graeca*, imported from Spain or North Africa. Reference is made to instances occurring in the United States, in spite of strict control of the trade in tortoises, in Chapter 13. Some years ago, when I was pathologist at the London Zoo, I was requested to supply information about possible respiratory pathogens carried by tortoises which could infect human beings. Research into the archives revealed that a number of organisms, including pneumococci, had been isolated from tortoises. The information was required by the government of the time to enable a reply to be given to a parliamentary question. The answer given in parliament was that no evidence existed that tortoises were ever infected with respiratory pathogens, which could be infective to man!

Birds

Wild birds, as we have seen, are important reservoirs of the influenzas and of arboviruses. They also suffer from enteric diseases caused by salmonellae, especially *Salmonella typhimurium*. Apart from the influenzas, their respiratory pathogens are different from those of man, except for psittacosis, which is undoubtedly the most important of the avian zoonoses.

A disease, which came to be known as psittacosis from the Greek word for parrot, was known to cause severe and often fatal pneumonia in man before the end of the last century. At that time, it was supposed to be associated only with parrots, but latterly its wide host range has become known and the term ornithosis is widely substituted for psittacosis. This is an unnecessary and pedantic change, which has led to confusion; some workers use psittacosis for the disease in whatever host, some ornithosis, while others call the disease in parrots or when derived from parrots psittacosis, in other birds or derived from other birds ornithosis. The term psittacosis has priority and will be used here whatever the context. Psittacosis is a disease primarily of birds, by which man is easily infected and to which he is very susceptible. It is caused by a microorganism, *Chlamydia psittaci*, which is transmitted by aerosol in dried faeces or feather dust. The organism is closely related to the rickettsias; there is only one other chlamydia known at present, *C. trachomatis*, which causes the eye disease of trachoma and Lymphogranuloma Venereum.

The chlamydia of psittacosis are found as harmless commensals in a wide variety of avian hosts, which are listed by Keymer (1974). Human cases can arise from any infected bird and virtually all groups of birds can carry infection. However, the human disease is far more severe when derived from psittacine birds than from other groups. The reason for this is not clear, though it is supposed that psittacines shed more of the infecting agent and so transmit a higher initial dose. Psittacosis, although it had been known for so long, came into prominence in 1930 when outbreaks occurred in many parts of the world. The outbreaks were associated with imported parrots chiefly from South America, and a great many deaths occurred amongst persons handling the birds both in the exporting and importing countries. In the United Kingdom and the United States, the importation of parrots was prohibited and the disease diminished both in the number of cases reported and in virulence. At this time, it was found also in Australia that both budgerigars and cockatoos were widely infected both in captivity and in the wild. In Europe and America, infection was found to be widespread in domestic aviaries and associated with outbreaks both in birds and man. Restrictions on the importation of parrots to Britain were lifted in 1951, but the increase of psittacosis cases was so great that they were reimposed in 1953. The same increase was experienced in the United States, when their ban was similarly lifted between 1951 and 1954.

There is, therefore, a clear association between the numbers of the larger parrots imported and the incidence and virulence of psittacosis. However, a ban on the importation of parrots does not mean the end of psittacosis as a disease of man, because reservoirs exist in wild, cage and farm birds. In wild birds, the most important reservoir is that of pigeons, which infest most towns and cities; it is believed that as many as 80% of town pigeons may carry infection, which may easily be passed to man in dried faeces or feather dust blown by the wind. There are also cases in which infection has been traced to garden birds, which at certain times of the year tap on windows and deposit their excreta on window sills. Amongst farm birds, the main culprits are turkeys which commonly carry infection and can pass it to those who handle them. Fortunately, psittacosis contracted from these sources is far less virulent than the parrot transmitted disease.

An important reservoir of psittacosis resides in budgerigars, of which there are estimated to be some five and a half million in Britain alone. Some are kept in isolated cages in living rooms or kitchens; some are in free flight aviaries; yet others are kept under so-called "homing" conditions. The latter fly around at liberty all day, but are encouraged to return to the aviary at night for food and shelter. Homing budgerigars come in contact with wild birds, particularly pigeons; even if initially free from psittacosis, they will inevitably become infected in the course of time. Even without the introduction of psittacosis from external sources, the disease can be self-perpetuating in budgerigar flocks.

The eradication of psittacosis would appear to be impossible. The elimination of all parrots, budgerigars and town pigeons would no doubt reduce its incidence to the point of being a rare disease. However, such drastic measures would not be tolerated by the public, and would in any case be socially undesirable. It does appear, however, that the ban on importation of parrots should be maintained, and homing budgerigars should be disallowed. Disease free stocks of budgerigars could no doubt be bred. Meanwhile, the numbers of pigeons in towns and cities should be controlled within reasonable limits. Fortunately, *Ch. psittaci* are sensitive to tetracycline therapy so that, although some resistant strains have appeared, most cases of psittacosis can be successfully treated when diagnosed. It would appear that the disease is often not diagnosed, and the medical profession could reasonably be alerted to the possibility that pneumonia cases may be due to psittacosis.

Rodents and Lagomorphs (rabbits and hares)

Pets, such as rabbits, mice, rats, guinea pigs and hamsters should only be acquired from reliable sources, and known to be free from human pathogens. When bred in captivity in sanitary surroundings, they should be safe pets for children provided that their food is kept free from contamination with rodent and bird faeces. If kept in outside runs, they should also somehow be kept from contact with wild birds and rodents. Exotic rodents, such as rats, mice, voles, lemmings and gerbils frequently carry a number of very unpleasant diseases, amongst which may be numbered plague, tularaemia, pseudotuberculosis, leptospirosis, salmonellosis and a number of other pathogens. A new and deadly disease, which has caused a number of deaths, has recently come into prominence, namely "Lassa Fever"; it is acquired from contact with a common African Rodent, the Multimammate Mouse (*Mastomys cricetus*). The disease is discussed further in Chapter 13.

Other Imported or Wild Animals

Hedgehogs are sometimes affected with human scabies, but seem otherwise to be quite safe as pets. When they become sick in captivity, it is usually due to faulty feeding. Unless provided with plenty of lime as in whole snails of which they are very fond, they develop rickets and die from pneumonia because of contraction of the chest cavity. There is no danger of cross-infection. Skunks are often sold as pets after their stink glands have been removed surgically. Since these animals are amongst the few known silent carriers of rabies, they cannot be recommended as safe pets. Apart perhaps from hedgehogs, fish and frogs, no animal captured in the wild can be recommended as a pet. Almost any such could be affected with toxoplasmosis, but dangers of cross-infection are not so great as with cats.

Dogs and Cats

Dogs and cats in their millions are the beloved inmates of British homes. Dogs have been the companions of man since the Stone Age, and cats at least since the days of the pharaohs. Yet it is only within the past twenty years that serious suggestions have been made that they could be inimical to human health. The indictment rests mainly on four zoonoses, all of which can have serious consequences. These are: — (i) hydatid; (ii) larva migrans; (iii) toxoplasmosis; and (iv) leukaemia.

Helminth Infections

Of hydatid enough has been said; the natural history of the disease is well understood and remedial measures can easily be taken.

Larva migrans, on the other hand, require some further scrutiny; the position has been well summarised by Woodruff (1969). Interest in the dangers of the migrating larvae of *Toxocara canis* in children was aroused by the report of Woodruff *et al.* (1961) of the case of a young boy, whose death was ascribed to this cause. Ensuing investigations showed that 20% of dogs in the London area were infected with *T. canis*; the question arose as to why, in view of the obviously large reservoir of *T. canis* and *T. cati* and the close contacts of dogs and cats with man, so few human cases were reported. The reported cases appeared to be confined to those in which the loss of sight in an eye from larva migrans rendered the diagnosis unmistakeable; it was argued that, if the worm reached the eye in some cases, infection of other organs, such as liver, spleen or even brain must be far more common. The development of a specific skin test for *Toxocara* made further investigation possible. Meanwhile, the death of a child from paralytic poliomyelitis had been described by Beautyman and Wolf (1951), in which a toxocaral larval granuloma was found in the brain, identified as due to *T. canis*. It was supposed that the worm larva might have carried a large dose of poliomyelitis virus from the gut to the brain. In consequence, the toxocara skin test was applied to a group of normal healthy persons, and to a group of persons who had suffered from paralytic poliomyelitis. The tests showed that toxocara infection had occurred seven times more frequently in those who had suffered from paralytic poliomyelitis than in those who had not. There is thus prima facie evidence that toxocara larvae may be an agent in the distribution of poliomyelitis virus through the body; they could be responsible for the spread of other infections also.

The investigation was then extended to persons suffering from epilepsy. Results in this case were not so convincing. All the same, the skin test for toxocara was positive $3\frac{1}{2}$ times more frequently in epileptics than in non-epileptics. It was concluded that some epileptic patients developed the condition as a result of toxocara larvae invading the brain and creating a focus of irritation there. Woodruff suggested further that *T. cati* might be one vehicle for the distribution of *Toxoplasma* within the body. Evidently, the synergistic role of larva migrans in distributing pathogens through the body has been insufficiently investigated.

These reports may seem alarming; tragic as they are, cases of severe disability or death from these canine and feline parasites are very few. Owing to the strange life history of *T. canis* in dogs, elimination of the parasite would be difficult or impossible to achieve, because the worms are encysted in the tissues. However, it is the suckling bitches and the puppies which are dangerous. Children should be kept away from bitches when suckling, and from puppies until they are some five months old; at the same time both bitch and puppies should be regularly dosed so as to eliminate the worms from the bowel. All excreta should be buried or burnt. Cats should be dosed at regular intervals, so as to keep them free from toxocara infection. If only the facts were better known both by doctors and parents, this problem could become of very small importance.

Toxoplasmosis

Toxoplasmosis is an ever present danger where cats are kept. The discovery of the life history of the parasite, described by Beverley

(1974), is so recent that its full implications have not been evaluated. However, reliable methods exist for serological diagnosis of infection and treatment is effective. The greatest problem again appears to arise from a lack of awareness amongst parents and medical practitioners of the prevalence and possible importance of *Toxoplasma*. Possibly cats should be regularly treated; the subject does not appear to have been studied. In cases of unidentified mild illness or irrational behaviour in children, tests for toxoplasma infection should be made and treatment given, if necessary. There could even be a case for routine testing of school children at an age when the infection was likely to cause problems.

Leukaemia

As to whether domestic animals play any part in the transmission of cancer viruses to man cannot be said. Feline leukaemia is of known viral origin, and statistics seem to show that the incidence of leukaemia is higher in children of families where cats are kept. Children should certainly be kept away from sick cats, especially if they are suffering from leukaemia.

Farm Animals

Diseases are acquired from farm animals from direct or indirect contact with them or from consumption of or handling their products. Today dangers of contracting disease from the consumption of animal products are infinitesimal compared with even a generation ago. Animals destined for slaughter for meat come from herds and flocks that have been subject to veterinary supervision; they are inspected by a veterinary surgeon before slaughter and the meat is inspected before being passed as fit for human consumption. Under such conditions, it is most unusual for meat that is in any way dangerous to be offered for sale. At the same time, milk is derived from dairy herds that are routinely inspected and maintained free from contagious abortion, tuberculosis and mastitis. Methods of milking and bottling are hygienic, and for greater safety the milk is pasteurised. Dangers from contagious abortion, tuberculosis, anthrax, tapeworm, trichinellosis should all be things of the past. It is, however, unavoidable that some animals, carrying or infected with salmonellae, should slip through the net and in this sphere, as we have seen, dangers of contracting infection from meat products have increased because of newer methods of handling food products; this is truest of poultry. Enough has been said of this elsewhere, and cases to illustrate the point are quoted in Chapter 13.

What is true of domestic products is not true of imported goods. The most obvious dangers are those already discussed in eggs or egg powders imported from the far east. A particularly serious source of danger exists in imported hides, which frequently carry spores of anthrax, and are a danger to tannery workers and to members of the public who may acquire goods, such as native drums, made from uncured skins. Anthrax spores may also be present in animal feeds, such as bone meal. In the past, tannery effluents have been responsible for contaminating pastures and, although this rarely happens today, great care is needed. Investigations showed that in 1958 nearly 25% of dry hides imported into Britain were contaminated with anthrax spores, and in 1959 18 of 21 samples of bone meal from Asian countries were similarly contaminated. Instances are quoted in Chapter 13 of enteric diseases contracted in the United States from cheese and other milk products bought in Mexico.

In today's western world, persons at greatest risk from farm animals and their products are those who work with them, such as farmers and veterinary surgeons, and those engaged in preparing and processing the carcasses. The risks arise from rickettsial diseases, such as Q Fever, from fungal and related diseases, such as ringworm, actinomyces, histoplasmosis, cryptococcosis and candidiasis, from bacterial diseases, such as tularaemia, listeriosis, vibriosis, salmonellosis and general septic conditions. Toxoplasmosis can be acquired from sheep, and poultry and rabbits can also be dangerous. Even so, the improvement in the general health of livestock has greatly reduced these risks also and a greater understanding of health hazards enables such persons largely to avoid risks of infections.

In countries, where the control of farm animal diseases and of meat products is less far advanced, hazards to the public from animal products are similar to those which formerly existed in western societies. Such dangers exist not only for human but animal populations also. Britain is maintained free from Foot and Mouth Disease; whenever the disease appears, it is again eradicated by a ruthless policy of slaughter of all susceptible animals on farms where infection is found and on farms within a prescribed radius. The source of Foot and Mouth Disease is invariably traced to infected meat products, usually beef or bacon. In 1975, I spent three months on an advisory mission for the Department of Overseas Development in Pakistan at Lahore. When there, I was amazed at the problems facing the very efficient Punjab Veterinary Service and the members of the excellent Lahore Veterinary College. Not only was tuberculosis rampant both in the human and animal populations, but glanders was prevalent among the lean, upstanding ponies, which draw the colourful tonga carts. As a disease, glanders is almost forgotten in Europe having been eradicated many years ago. It is caused by the bacillus *Pfeiferella mallei*; it is serious in horses and in man causes a pneumonitis which is almost invariably fatal. The former British head of the Lahore Veterinary College, a well known veterinary surgeon, Dr. Gaiger, contracted infection while there and died of it. While foci of infections such as these continue to exist, there remains the danger that they could again be reintroduced to western countries under conditions in which they might not immediately be recognised. The price of freedom from such diseases is eternal vigilance.

Horses are perhaps the animals that are most moved around the world for purposes of racing and to acquire good breeding stock. Some years ago, a consignment of dwarf Argentine ponies was shipped from South America for the London Zoo. The ponies were refused admission to Britain, because the ship had been diverted to a West African port, and it was feared that they might have become infected with a mosquito-borne virus disease, African Horse Sickness. The authorities appear to have overlooked the far greater dangers that they might be infected with Equine Encephalitis, also transmitted by mosquitos. This danger could exist with any horses shipped from the American continent, as they frequently are for purposes of racing.

This chapter, as said, highlights some of the problems of man's relationship with his domestic animals. The dangers are not great and are diminished to small proportions with proper vigilance and sensible precautions. In the next chapter, we shall turn our attention to marine animals.

CHAPTER 12

Marine Animals

In many parts of the world seafoods provide the main source of high class protein, and at the present time nations are vying with each other for the right to exploit marine resources in a world in which reserves of high class protein are diminishing. Marine foods are acquired either from the open seas or from estuaries, rivers and fishponds. Most of it is in the form of fish, but a significant proportion is derived from invertebrate marine life, such as lobsters or crabs, or shellfish, oysters, clams, mussels and so on. Fish farming has been practised in the far east from time immemorial, and in the west oysters have been raised in oyster beds at least since Roman times. From time immemorial, man has been polluting the waters with his excreta and disjecta; it would be surprising if the marine environment did not contribute to his cycles of disease. They have certainly done so in the past, but dangers are today on the increase because of the industrial wastes that are introducing new hazards.

During our studies, we have seen that certain parasites rely for their transmission on secondary hosts that live in water. The tapeworm, *Diphyllobothrium latum*, is acquired by eating fish. Schistosomes are acquired from snails that live in water, as are many other trematodes. On the whole, sea water possesses remarkable powers of disinfection, and it is surprising how few outbreaks of enteric disease are attributed to eating seafoods. Crabs, in particular, live by scavenging the sea bed in areas where sewage is discharged, but are eaten all over the world with impunity. Shellfish, particularly the filter feeders such as oysters, clams and mussels, often acquire enteric organisms from contaminated water, concentrate them, and transmit infection. Oysters have been responsible for outbreaks of typhoid and paratyphoid. Even fish, such as the ubiquitous grey mullet, which feed by ingesting estuary mud, must theoretically be suspect.

Oysters and clams, as already seen, have been implicated in transmitting the virus of infectious hepatitis. Little confidence can be felt that, as the world's food resources diminish and populations increase, more diseases will not come to be spread in foods acquired from aquatic environments; the dangers will increase as the practice of farming aquatic environments spreads more widely. The ability of pathogens to become adapted to new modes of transmission is exemplified by the so-called "Salmon Poisoning" of dogs and foxes. This disease is a rare rickettsiosis, acquired by eating salmon. The intermediate host of the Rickettsia is a small trematode, which inhabits the gut of dogs or foxes; the larval form is found in salmon and infection of the main host occurs when the salmon is eaten. This is the only known rickettsia, of which the intermediate host is other than an arthropod. Other pathogens could become similarly adapted under conditions of intensive food culture in water. Already in the far east, a number of serious trematode infections are associated with fish-eating habits.

The impact of marine life on human health is further revealed in the so-called "red tide" phenomenon (Hutner *et al.* 1972). Red tides are caused by the "blooming" at certain times of pigmented micro-organisms, which live in the sea. This is an extraordinary phenomenon of marine ecology, in which two quite different forms of marine life are involved, the one blue-green algae, the other protozoal flagellates. The best known of the blue-green algae is *Trichodesmium erythraeum*, which is responsible for the name of the Red Sea; its sudden blooms often cover thousands of square miles of sea water. The blooms, resulting from *T. erythraeum*, and most other blue-green algae, are non-toxic; they have the power to fix nitrogen and probably play an important part in adding to the oceans' nitrogen stores. However, one group, *Microcystis*, is toxic and is blamed for causing a disease in South America, known as "ciguatera", acquired from eating fish which have fed on the algae. Red tides due to coloured flagellates also occur in sudden blooms, which may be of enormous extent. The organisms are extremely toxic and kill fish in enormous numbers either by toxicity or by reducing the oxygen content of the water. Persons walking along contaminated beaches develop allergic symptoms. If fish or shellfish, which have fed on the flagellates, are eaten, acute toxic symptoms result and death may occur. The condition may justifiably be regarded as a zoonosis, because it is a disease of fish which man acquires from eating them.

A more insidious danger from the consumption of seafoods arises where fish have consumed toxic chemicals and concentrated them. As Bourne (1972) and Johnston (1976) show, all noxious chemicals or radioactive wastes discharged into the rivers or the sea are a potential danger to human health. Such discharges, furthermore, become distributed globally throughout the seas in an unpredictable fashion. For example, DDT has been recovered in significant amounts from animals, such as penguins, which live solely in the Antarctic. The most notorious case of intoxication from a heavy metal is that of mercury, as described by Burton and Leatherhead (1971). Since this may doubtfully be regarded as a zoonosis, I shall confine discussion to this single problem in illustration.

A causal relationship between consumption of seafoods and mercury poisoning was first suspected in Japan, where some 137 persons died between 1954 and 1960 from eating shellfish contaminated with methyl mercury. The mercury came from effluents from a factory producing vinyl chloride and acetaldehyde. In Sweden also, fishing has had to be forbidden in some of the largest lakes because of mercury pollution, and in Australia the sale of school shark for human consumption has been forbidden for the same reason. In Britain, as discussed by Hicks (1975), fish caught in the Irish Sea show unacceptably high levels of mercury, resulting from discharges into Morecambe Bay from chlorine alkali works.

Discharges of mercury into the seas is mostly in the form of metallic mercury. Being both insoluble and heavy, the metal cannot contaminate the water and is harmless. Prima facie, therefore, the metal could not be damaging to human health, but for two circumstances. First, the metallic mercury falls to the bottom and becomes incorporated into the mud sediments; secondly, it is converted in the mud into an organic compound by a mud-living bacterium, the presence of which is due to pollution of the water by sewage. Even so, the concentration of methyl mercury in the bacteria is not sufficiently high as to be dangerous. The bacteria, however, are eaten by crustacea, which are themselves eaten by minnows. The minnows, in their turn, are eaten by larger fish, and the fish are caught and eaten by man. At each link of this food chain, the mercury becomes more concentrated, so that by the time it reaches the fish, which man eats, it has reached toxic levels. Furthermore, mercury is a cumulative poison, so that a toxic level is reached in time, if fish is an important article of diet. The chain of toxicity may be depicted as under: —

$\begin{cases} \text{Factory effluent (metallic mercury)} \\ \text{Sewage pollution (bacteria)} \end{cases}$ $\longrightarrow$ methyl mercury $\longrightarrow$ crustacea $\longrightarrow$ minnow $\longrightarrow$ fish.

Methyl mercury has a direct action on certain areas of the brain. The effects are not readily discernible as mercury poisoning and have been widely interpreted as mental defect. The gait becomes unsteady, vision is blurred and limited; there is deafness; the fingers and toes become numb. Affected persons suffer from a curious inability to conduct an intelligent conversation with more than one person at a time; they also suffer personality changes, such as excessive self-consciousness and embarrassment, timidity, anxiety and indecision; there is increased irritability with despondency and depression, and resentment of criticism. The symptoms develop slowly, so that an association with mercury poisoning becomes even more difficult to suspect.

Mercury is today a rare metal and world supplies are likely to be inadequate in the future. It is, therefore, nonsensical to discharge it into the water. It can easily be recovered from effluents, and provides a profitable sideline to other activities. Contamination of waters with mercury is, therefore, an activity, which must not be permitted to continue. Nevertheless, initially it appeared to be harmless; the lesson should be learned that potentially toxic substances should not be discharged into water under any circumstances. The story of mercury is given here as an example of the mounting dangers of these thoughtless discharges to a valuable food resource. Is this a zoonosis? In the author's opinion, it is. The greek words νοσος (nosos) or νοσημα (nosema) mean a pathological condition. They do not necessarily imply an infection, though the word zoonosis is usually used in this sense. Mercury poisoning in fish can, therefore, be rightly regarded as a zoonosis, illustrative of a branch of this study which is likely to become of greater importance.

CHAPTER 13

Selected Examples of Recent Zoonotic Incidents

Introduction

In this final chapter is quoted a selection of disease outbreaks, which have arisen in modern times as zoonoses, or which are potential zoonoses and emphasise some of the lessons to be learned about them. The cases cited have all been culled from "Morbidity and Mortality", a weekly publication of the US Department of Health, Education and Welfare — Center for Disease Control, Atlanta, Georgia. This work has been used in preference to reports from other areas, because it is unique. The excellence of disease investigation and reporting in the United States is unrivalled, and for geographical reasons the variety of conditions described is exceptionally wide. Moreover, where disease outbreaks have occurred in other countries which are of especial interest, these too are described.

In this work, we have studied three areas of zoonoses. First, we have considered those purely human diseases which must, in the past, have been derived from animal sources; secondly, we have considered diseases, which may be establishing themselves at the present time in human populations, and which are likely to have an animal origin — such as influenza A and cancer; thirdly, we have studied diseases, which currently affect human individuals and populations, and which are derived from animal sources. The present histories quoted are solely taken from the latter. Thus, the numerous reports in "Morbidity and Mortality" of influenza, measles and other such epidemics have been omitted. The order, in which these cases are arranged, is broadly that in which the subjects appear in the book.

Plague

It will be recalled that, whereas pandemic or epidemic pneumonic plague no longer occurs, there exist endemic plague foci in many parts of the world and that human cases occur sporadically as a result of transfer of infection from wildlife reservoirs. The situation in the United States was reported in "Morbidity and Mortality" 22:25 (June 23, 1973) as under: —

In 1970, a record number of 13 human bubonic plague cases associated with rural exposure was reported; two were detected in 1971, and one in 1972; none had been reported as of June 1st, 1973. Nevertheless, plague activity remained high among wild rodents in areas where human cases appeared in the past — Arizona, California, New Mexico, and Colorado. In 1973, plague epizootics were reported in wild rodents from three widely separated counties in California: Siskigon, Tulare, and Riverside. At Siskigon, the epizootic occurred in Wood Rats at Lava Beds National Monument, and forced its closure to visitors. In New Mexico, an epizootic occurred among Prairie Dogs near Shiprock, San Juan County, requiring vector control over 5000 acres to protect the resident Navajo population. This situation arose directly from an epizootic among prairie dogs in south west Colorado during 1971 and 1972.

Plague epizootics have been occurring among prairie dogs since 1963 in contiguous parts of north east Arizona, north west New Mexico, south west Colorado and south east Utah, a region known ecologically as the Navajonian Biome. Since 1963, 12 prairie dog associated cases have occurred in this region, mostly on the Navajo Indian Reservation. The problem in south west Colorado has been amplified by a great increase of prairie dogs on the west slopes of the Rocky Mountains in the past few years. These are all rural and wilderness areas; urban centres are not threatened.

A wild rodent plague epizootic, and its possible implications, is described in "Morbidity and Mortality" 23:29 (July 20th, 1974). On June 21st *Yersinia* (*Pasteurella*) *pestis* was isolated from *Peromyscus paniculatus* fleas at Moraine Camp Ground, Rocky Mountain National Park, which had to be closed to the public in consequence. There were very high populations of rodents, especially small ground squirrels (*Spermophilus richardsoni*) and chipmunks (*Eutamias spp.*), probably the result of feeding by visitors. These are all known to be susceptible to plague, and suffer high mortality during epizootics; they carry many fleas during the summer months. The camp site was treated with insecticidal dust, and the flea numbers on squirrels and chipmunks were reduced from 2·0 per animal to 0·8.

Seven human plague cases are described between July 1973 and October 1974. The report in "Morbidity and Mortality" 23:50 (December 14th, 1974) gives an account of plague in two cases in New Mexico resulting from direct and indirect contact with wild rabbits. In the first case, a woman had skinned a rabbit infested with fleas and developed bubonic plague. The rabbit was recovered from her freezer and was found to be positive for plague bacilli. In the second case, infection was contracted from one of the owner's cats, which one night slept on his bed; the cat had caught a rabbit and appears to have been harbouring temporarily rabbit fleas. Both these patients recovered with antibiotic therapy.

We will discuss one further plague case reported in "Morbidity and Mortality" 22:30 (July 28th, 1973). Between July 6th and 7th, a 9 year old girl from near Payson, Arizona, became ill with headache, fever and a swollen right axillary gland. Her blood was found to be infected with plague bacilli, and she was treated and recovered. She appeared to have acquired the infection near the family's mountain home. Plague bacilli were found in the animals of this area in February 1972, when another plague case had resulted from contact with a wild lynx. At that time, a serological survey had been made of the wild carnivore populations and widespread plague activity was found on the Coconino Plateau and in contiguous, ecologically similar areas immediately north of the site where this case was apparently contracted.

Enteric Infections

The point has been made that, whereas the incidence of most infectious diseases has diminished in modern times because of advances in medical science, that of enteric disease has tended to increase. This is associated with newer ways of preparing and storing food. The mortality associated with these diseases is not usually high, because they are readily controlled by antibiotic therapy. They can, on the other hand, cause great inconvenience or spoil an expensive holiday on a cruise ship. They could be dangerous, if, as sometimes happens, they should occur on a long distance flight. For this reason, it is usually arranged that the crew eat different food from the passengers, and that the two co-pilots also eat separate meals. It is said that the commonest cause of outbreaks of food poisoning is failure to refrigerate properly meals that have been prepared in advance, and keeping them too long at ambient or warm-up temperatures. There is no doubt truth in this, but at some stage, the food has become contaminated with a pathogen, and these faulty procedures merely give it the opportunity to multiply.

The organisms most commonly incriminated in enteric zoonoses are salmonellae, followed by staphylococci. The main vehicles are contaminated milk or milk products and infected meat. Shellfish are also responsible for the transmission of enteric pathogens and of the virus of infectious hepatitis; they also transmit an organism of the cholera group, which is free-living in inshore waters and causes serious disease.

Staphylococcal Food Poisoning

We shall start by describing two cases of staphylococcal food-borne infections. The staphylococcus usually involved is *Staphylococcus aureus*, which manufactures a powerful toxin. For this reason, outbreaks tend to be rapid in onset and very violent. They are usually the result of a septic injury on the hand of the food preparer, but can also arise from an infected food product, as is shown in the case below, from "Morbidity and Mortality" 23:17 (April 27th, 1974): —

During some five weeks, episodes of illness compatible with staphylococcal food poisoning were reported, which were associated with the consumption of milkshakes prepared from milkshake mixes. The mixes were prepared by two independent Pennsylvania dairies. There occurred nine separate episodes of acute gastrointestinal illness involving at least 45 persons in Chester and York Counties. The chief symptoms were nausea and vomiting; the median incubation period was six hours and duration 20 hours. The mixes came from dairy A. Associated with mixes from dairy B, there were 37 episodes involving approximately 120 people from Chester, Lackawanna, Delaware, Montgomery, Lehigh and Philadelphia Counties in Pennsylvania; Camden, Gloucester and Mercer Counties in New Jersey; Allegheny and Garrett Counties in Maryland; and Mineral and Hardy Counties in West Virginia.

When the milkshakes were withdrawn by the dairies, the nuisance ceased. Both dairies used whey as an ingredient of their milkshake mixes; both obtained their whey from a common source. A sample of the whey was obtained and found to be contaminated with coagulase-positive staphylococci with enterotoxigenic properties.

The second case to be quoted at length involves eggs and highlights the dangers of such outbreaks, when they occur on aircraft on long distance flights. Outbreaks were reported on three such flights on the same day, two scheduled flights and one charter flight, originating in southern Europe and destined for the United States. These are reported in "Morbidity and Mortality" 22:46 (November 17th, 1973): —

On the first flight, passengers suffered from severe gastrointestinal symptoms 1-2 hours after eating a meal taken on board in Lisbon. On arrival in New York, 35 of 47 sick passengers were medically examined and released; two of the passengers suffered from severe prostration and were admitted to hospital; the remaining 10 were detained overnight for observation. The second flight was similarly involved, 50 of the 91 passengers being affected. Several of the older passengers became cyanotic and required oxygen, and a four year old boy became hypotensive. After arrival at San Juan, eight patients were admitted to hospital and required to be given fluids intravenously. Stools of two of the patients yielded *Staphylococcus aureus* on culture. On the charter flight, the incubation period was shorter, from ½ to 2 hours, and 150 of 179 passengers were affected.

The source of the infection was traced to a *Staphylococcus aureus* contaminated dessert — "Custard Bavarois". This was made from egg yolk, sugar, milk, gelatine, chocolate, gooseberry juice and strawberry jelly. In its preparation, there were several pouring and chilling steps in a four hour period. It was then packed into individual passenger trays and refrigerated in a holding area for 2½ hours until the plane was provisioned. The temperature of the holding area was found to be 62°F. and had been so for several weeks. For flight 3, the holding time was 2½ hours longer.

Streptococcal Food Poisoning

Streptococci are usually associated with respiratory complaints and are usually transmitted by airborne infection. That they too can be transmitted in food is shown by the following report from "Morbidity and Mortality" 23:43 (October 26th, 1974): —

Beta haemolytic streptococcal pharyngitis attacked 320 of 690 inmates of the County Jail in Miami. The source of the infection was an egg salad prepared by a prison officer with pharyngitis. The food had been prepared in advance and was improperly refrigerated. In this outbreak, the food was merely a vehicle for transmitting disease from one human being to another. It is not, therefore, a zoonosis, but illustrated a principle, as does the following involving *Bacillus cereus* in food-poisoning outbreaks in England and Wales, quoted from "Morbidity and Mortality" 22:42 (October 20th, 1973): —

Bacillus Cereus *Food Poisoning*

There were 18 reports of food poisoning in the United Kingdom, in which 12 Chinese restaurants and "take-away" shops and one health food store were involved. The source was fried or boiled rice. The rice was prepared in the usual Chinese way. Large quantities are boiled, then left at room temperature from 12 hours to three days. The rice is then either reheated (boiled rice) or fried for a short time with freshly beaten egg (fried rice). The total number taken ill was 57 and *Bacillus cereus* was isolated from 32. The incubation period was from 15 minutes to 11 hours, mostly 1½ to 4½ hours. Nausea and vomiting were the predominant symptoms. *B. cereus* was isolated from a number of uncooked rice grains. The spores survive boiling and the vegetative cells in the boiled rice stored at ambient temperatures readily grow and multiply. Restaurant owners are reluctant to refrigerate boiled rice because the grains stick together, making it difficult to toss them together with the beaten egg during frying. This again shows how a pathogen may multiply in a prepared food, if it is kept too long at temperatures suitable for its growth. *Bacillus cereus* is not zoonotic, but the same principles apply in the case of the salmonelloses, case reports of which will be studied next. Of the dysenteries, caused by shigellae, only one instance is quoted of a human outbreak from an animal source ("Morbidity and Mortality" 22:19 of May 12th, 1973) when the source of infection was non-human primates.

Salmonelloses

Eighteen cases of salmonella outbreaks have been culled from the pages of "Morbidity and Mortality". A large number of species of salmonella have been involved. Of these cases, no less than six have resulted from direct contact with "turtles", by which is usually meant tortoises or terrapins. These animals are widely kept in the United States as pets. They are bred in very large numbers on "turtle" farms, of which one in Mississippi ships many thousands annually to other states of the Union. It is a legal requirement that all turtles shipped across State borders must have a certificate that they are free of the main human pathogens that they carry, namely organisms of the salmonella and Arizona groups; federal regulations prescribe how the tests are to be done, and there is no suggestion that they are not conscientiously performed. Nevertheless, most of the turtle-associated salmonella infections have arisen from certified turtles, and it would appear that these reptiles can be no more rendered free from salmonella than mammals can be rendered free of coliform bacilli. The following is the report published in "Morbidity and Mortality" 23:24 (June 15th, 1974) describing the situation relating to turtle-associated salmonellosis following the first year of operation of new regulations regarding certification of interstate shipments: —

During 1973, 184 isolations were made from turtles or turtle water as against a mean of 200 per year for the previous five years. Of these 27% were the result of investigations into 35 bacteriologically confirmed human cases. Between December 1972 and February 1974, 39 lots, containing 474 000 turtles, were certified as free from salmonella and Arizona infection. The turtles originated from five sources in Mississippi and Louisiana; salmonella were isolated from 15 (38%) of the 39 certified lots. The organisms isolated were *Salmonella panama,*

S. braenderup, S. litchfield, S. typhimurium. In eight associated human cases, the organisms involved were *S. braenderup, S. litchfield* and *S. typhimurium.* We may quote at length one particularly serious case, in which the patient developed meningitis as a result of the salmonella infection — "Morbidity and Mortality" 23:14 (April 6th, 1974): —

A one month old infant was admitted to hospital in Cincinatti, Ohio, with a one day history of fever, anorexia and severe lethargy. *S. enteritidis* was isolated both from the stool and from the cerebro-spinal fluid. The child was treated with antibiotics for 10 days and became afebrile and alert. One week later the baby was readmitted, because of a recurrence of fever, severe lethargy and the occurrence of three generalised convulsions. Spinal fluid was again purulent and blood and spinal fluid again grew *S. enteritidis.* After two weeks of intravenous chloramphenicol therapy, the baby was again alert and afebrile, but a further relapse occurred three days later and purulent spinal fluid again grew salmonella. It was eventually necessary for intraventricular and intravenous chloramphenicol to be administered for six weeks, before there was permanent recovery.

The family owned two pet turtles purchased one year prior to the baby's illness. Both turtles had positive anal swabs for *S. enteritidis.* The baby had no direct contact with the turtles, but his sibs 2 and 4 years old, often played with the turtles and also had frequent contact with the infant. The rest of the family remained healthy, except for the father, who became ill with acute salmonella gastro-enteritis shortly after the baby.

Turkey-associated salmonellosis was reported in "Morbidity and Mortality" 23:3 (January 19th, 1974). On Friday, November 30th, 1973, and extending over the weekend, some 468 of 891 high school students at Grundy, Virginia, suffered from vomiting and diarrhoea, 70 were sent to hospital. They all eventually recovered. Stool specimens from 10 students and staff members were found positive for *Salmonella reading.* Turkey salad was implicated as the source of infection. Eighteen turkeys had been stored on November 21st, 12 having been cooked on November 19th and boned on the 20th. The other six were cooked overnight on November 20th, and boned at about 8.30 the next morning. All the turkeys were kept warm in a large serving pan until served at 1.00 p.m. The latter six turkeys were not served, but stored in the refrigerator. All the kitchen staff had taken a hand in preparing the turkeys.

Two of the kitchen staff took some of the unserved turkey home and fed it to their families who became violently ill with fever, vomiting and diarrhoea within twelve hours of eating it. The turkey at that time was not suspected, though one affected person was found in the third week of December with a stool positive for *S. reading*. However, on November 28th and 29th, the frozen turkey was placed in the refrigerator to thaw. By 8.00 a.m. it was still frozen, and so was placed in roasting pans for about twenty minutes. It was then put through a meat chopper at 10.00 a.m. and mixed with chopped boiled eggs, chopped pickles and salad dressing. One woman, who ate some of the turkey from the roasting pans later became ill with typical symptoms of salmonellosis. *S. reading* had apparently multiplied to a concentration to cause illness before the unused turkey was refrozen on November 21st.

One more case will be quoted at length. A series of salmonella outbreaks, in which broiler chickens were involved occurred in Britain and was described in "Morbidity and Mortality" 22:3 (June 9th, 1973). The organism responsible was *Salmonella virchow*, a species uncommon in Britain before 1967. There was an annual average of 11 reported cases for the five years 1962-1966. In 1967, 1968, and 1969, the figures were 51, 229 and 361. In 1967 and 1968, most isolations came from the north west, and there was a large outbreak in the Liverpool area. The infection came from broiler chickens from one particular packing station. Further cases followed in the Midlands, and one outbreak caused the closure of a maternity unit. The mother, who introduced the infection, had eaten chicken from this same station. In 1969, the human cases were again concentrated in the north west, but spread also to southern counties. From 1970 to 1972, cases diminished, but *S. virchow* continued to be isolated from poultry, especially broilers.

Botulism

One of the commonest causes of fatalities from canned foods is botulism, but this can rarely be described as a zoonosis. One instance, however, where this term might be applied is described in "Morbidity and Mortality" 23:47 (November 23rd, 1974). A man and his wife, living in Alaska, suffered from severe symptoms of botulism, from which they were narrowly rescued by heroic hospital treatment. The disease resulted from eating salmon dipped in seal oil. The salmon had been caught one month earlier and dried in the sun. The seal oil was derived from a dead, partially decomposed seal 7-10 days earlier. Botulinus E toxin was recovered from seal meat, which had been stored, but not from the oil, which, however, contained particles of meat.

Infectious Hepatitis

Infectious Hepatitis, as is now well known, is commonly contracted from contact with newly imported primates. One such case is reported in "Morbidity and Mortality" 22:49 (December 8th, 1973), in which five persons at an Ohio zoo were infected by a shipment of three siamangs, the first time that these apes, allied to gibbons, have been incriminated. Hepatitis A can also be water-borne and a case is described in "Morbidity and Mortality" 22:14 (April 7th, 1973), in which nine cases occurred in different families from drinking contaminated water from two surface springs in Alabama. In this way, shellfish can become infected and pass the virus to persons who eat them. One such case is reported in "Morbidity and Mortality" 22:46 (November 17th, 1973) and is worth recording *in extense*: —

In a 17 day period from September 20th to October 6th, 1973, some 265 clinical cases of hepatitis A were identified as resulting from the consumption of raw oysters. The majority of the cases occurred in Houston, Texas, where 250 persons were affected after eating at nine different restaurants. A further episode occurred in Georgia, where 15 of 150 persons contracted the disease after attending a seafood dinner on September 21st. All of the implicated oysters seemed to have originated from a single Louisiana supplier. Distribution of the suspect oysters was traced to six states, Texas, Louisiana, Alabama, Georgia, Florida and Tennessee. Investigations in these states revealed an additional 39 cases of hepatitis associated with eating raw shellfish.

Vibriosis

A different form of infectious enteric disease derived from seafood is that caused by *Vibrio parahaemolyticus*, related to the cholera germ. This organism lives its natural life in inshore waters and often infects shellfish, including oysters, crab, lobster and shrimp. A survey of the situation in the United States between 1969 and 1972 is given in "Morbidity and Mortality" 22:27 (July 7th, 1973): —

There were 13 outbreaks of gastro-enteritis attributed to *Vibrio parahaemolyticus* in the period 1969 to 1972; these reports came from Pacific and Gulf coast states and from Hawaii. Approximately, 1200 persons became ill in 13 outbreaks. The attack rates varied from 24% to 88% with a mean of 51%. Most cases were in adults, but no pattern of susceptibility by age group or sex was noted, nor was there any evidence of spread among family members. Incubation periods ranged from 4 to 96 hours, with means of 15 to 24 hours. All the outbreaks were attributed to infected shellfish.

Diarrhoea was the dominant symptom (80-100%), described as watery and explosive; there were no bloody or mucoid stools. Abdominal cramps, nausea and vomiting were frequent; headache infrequent. Fever with or without chills was described in about a quarter of the cases. The duration of the illness ranged from several hours to more than 10 days, with a median period of 72 hours. No severe complications or deaths were reported. Crab, shrimp, lobster and oysters were incriminated as the sources of infection. Though most of the food was eaten cooked, inadequate cooking and refrigeration had been blamed. Results of these investigations are similar to those obtained among hundreds of outbreaks in Japan, where the seafood is mostly eaten raw.

Tularaemia

Of other bacterial diseases, that most frequently reported is tularaemia. "Morbidity and Mortality" 23:42 (October 19th, 1974) reported the disease in a boy, who suffered from tick bites when on vacation on Martha's Vineyard Island; in this case, there was no direct contact with rodents. A typical case is reported in "Morbidity and Mortality" 23:16 (April 20th, 1974). Two persons became infected, a woman of 61 and her son aged 36. The mother was treated and recovered, but her son died. The woman's son, together with his son and brother-in-law had killed six rabbits on a hunting trip. The patient who died had skinned and eviscerated the rabbits, while three of the six rabbits were cooked and eaten by the mother.

One further case is worthy of detailed mention, which occurred in an endemic plague area and diagnosis was obscured because the symptoms and history resembled those of plague. The case is described in "Morbidity and Mortality" 23:34 (August 24th, 1974). A 39 year old man from Coolidge, New Mexico, developed rhinorrhoea, headache, general malaise and fever of 103°F. His condition showed improvement until May 24th, when a tender swelling developed at the anterior axillary line. On June 6th, he had a rectal swelling and widespread tender swellings of lymph nodes. Aspirates from lymph nodes failed to reveal suspicious organisms and were negative for plague bacilli with fluorescent antibody. Cultures of blood, sputum and aspirate were also negative. However, agglutination and haemagglutinin tests showed the presence of tularaemia infection. The diagnosis was made the more difficult, because the patient denied having suffered from recent insect or tick bites, or having had a tick bite carbuncle. He denied also having skinned or dressed rabbits or other small mammals. He and his wife, however, had eaten prairie dog meat well cooked. The symptoms and history of this disease occurring in an enzootic plague area suggested bubonic plague, whereas it was in fact a glandular form of tularaemia. In the area involved, prairie dog fleas have been found infected with *Francisella (Pasteurella) tularensis*.

Brucellosis

Some interesting cases of brucellosis associated with the consumption of Mexican cheese are reported in "Morbidity and Mortality" 22:23 (June 9th, 1973). The first outbreak occurred on February 19th, 1973. A 24 year old woman was admitted to hospital in Denver, Colorado, with a three week history of fever, chills, and generalised abdominal and low back pain. She was found to have a rectal temperature of 40·9°C., tachycardia, soft systolic murmur at the cardiac base, mild lower quadrant abdominal tenderness, hepatosplenomegaly and bilateral costovertebral angle tenderness. The haematocrit was 28%, Haemoglobin 8·4 gm%, and there was evidence of disseminated intravascular coagulation without bleeding. Brucella agglutination titres were 1:3 200 and blood was positive for *Brucella melitensis.* The patient recovered with antibiotic therapy. On March 13th, her 24 year old sister was also admitted to hospital with similar but milder symptoms. Brucella agglutination in her case was 1:320. She too recovered with treatment. Three other members of the household escaped infection. The mother-in-law of the second patient had purchased goat cheese at a market in Juarez, Mexico. This was plainly the source of infection, though it was eaten by several members of the two families with impunity. Four other cases of *Br. melitensis* infection occurred at this same time in El Paso, Texas, two of which were also traced to cheese bought in Juarez market.

Brucellosis in the United States occurs mostly in workers in the livestock industry and in meat processing. In recent years, about 15% of cases have been associated with the ingestion of presumably unpasteurised dairy products. Of the 190 cases reported in 1971, 19 were associated with Mexican cheese or dairy products, and two persons contracted the disease from Italian dairy products.

Tuberculosis

A case of tuberculosis contracted from a pet monkey was reported in "Morbidity and Mortality" 22:17 (April 28th, 1973), which should serve as an object lesson to persons considering keeping monkeys as pets. On October 23rd, 1972, a pet stump-tailed macaque monkey (*Macaca arctoides*) was tuberculin tested because of persistent cough, and found positive. On X-ray, nodular lesions were found in the right lung, and at autopsy granulomatous lesions were found in the lungs, liver, spleen and one lymph node. *Mycobacterium tuberculosis* was isolated from the lungs. All five members of the family were tuberculin tested on October 31st, and found negative. However, in December the 9 year old son was positive and the 18 year old daughter in January 1973.

On investigation an unusual and interesting case history was revealed. The monkey had been bought by the Washington family on October 9th, 1972. Before this, the monkey had been kept by several different California residents. It was one of two stump-tails (A and B) purchased by two different individuals from an Inglewood, California, pet shop in 1969. In March 1971, both monkeys were sold to a third person, who had been admitted to hospital with active tuberculosis in May 1970 with a sputum positive for *M. tuberculosis*. At the time monkeys A and B were purchased, he had a third stump-tail, which he had bought as an infant in early 1970. When the owner went to hospital, monkey C was tested for tuberculosis but was negative. On retesting in August and October 1970, C was tuberculin positive and had a positive chest X-ray; the owner, however, refused to dispose of it. From March to November 1971, the three monkeys were housed in the same outdoor cage. In November, monkeys A and B were boarded at the home of another family. Monkey C died of tuberculosis on March 18th, 1972 and *M. tuberculosis* was isolated from the tissues. Monkey B died in June 1972 of undetermined causes; no necropsy was performed, but there was a history of persistent cough. Monkey A was later sold to the Washington family. Evidently monkey C caught tuberculosis from the owner and infected A and B. A then infected the Washington owner.

Anthrax

A serious outbreak of anthrax was reported in "Morbidity and Mortality" 23:39 (September 28th, 1974), which fortunately affected only animals at a private game park, near Sequoia, Washington. Forty-two deaths occurred among 125 carnivores, mostly cougars and other large felines. The anthrax was traced to a horse, which had been fed to the animals; it had evidently died of anthrax. The horse had been on a trip to the mountains and had carried a pack saddle, which was stuffed with goat hair from Pakistan and Afghanistan. The hair was shown to carry anthrax spores.

Another anthrax incident, in which human beings were involved, was described in "Morbidity and Mortality" 23:16 and 17 (April 20th and 27th, 1974). Infection was attributed to Haitian drums and occurred in this way. On December 28th, 1973, a navy journalist photographer assigned to a hospital ship, suffered irritation in her left eye, and attributed it to her contact lens. Next morning she had painless oedema of the upper left eyelid. In 24 hours, the swelling increased and the lid became slightly inflamed. By December 30th, the eye was completely closed by the swelling, which extended laterally to the side of the face and to her forehead. In spite of treatment with hot packs and antibiotics, the swelling continued to increase and there was pain around the eye, smears from which revealed *Bacillus anthracis*. Although penicillin therapy was then given, the patient was admitted to hospital on December 31st because of deterioration of the symptoms, and the upper eyelid had become bluish-black. The temperature was 101°F. Eventual recovery took place. Scarring persisted, so that she cannot close her left eyelid.

On November 8th, the patient had boarded the hospital ship, which was en route for Haiti, at the Panama Canal. In Port au Prince, she bought seven wooden drums which had goat hide drumheads with a fringe of hair intact. At this time, ship's personnel treated about forty cases of anthrax in Haiti residents, but the patient had no contact with them. The ship arrived in Florida on December 15th. The weekend before Christmas, the patient sent three drums to her parents in Louisiana and two to friends in Michigan; she kept two drums herself. *B. anthracis* was isolated from one of the Michigan drums, one from the Louisiana drums, and one of the drums kept in Florida.

Relapsing Fever

There is one report of Relapsing Fever cases in Georgia and Arizona — "Morbidity and Mortality" 22:29 (July 21st, 1973). These cases are described as direct man - tick - man transmission cycles; the possible existence of wildlife reservoirs, as in opossums, is not mentioned. Little is known of this, but it is probable that such wildlife reservoirs do exist, as discussed by me in "Zoonoses of Primates" (1967). The reports are as under: —

On June 22nd, 1973, a 12 year old girl from Atlanta, Georgia, became ill with chills, headache, and fever (104°F.) which lasted three days. After the fever subsided the girl felt completely well, but on July 4th, she had a febrile episode of two days' duration. On July 11th she was examined, found to be normal, and no therapy was given. On July 12th, her temperature rose briefly to 104°F. On July 19th, she had another episode of fever and went back to the doctor, who found loosely coiled spirochaetes in blood smears at the time she was febrile. She was treated with tetracycline. The patient had visited several western national parks with her parents between June 17th and 21st.

On June 18th, they had stayed in an old wooden cabin on the North Rim of the Grand Canyon; neither the girl nor her family could recall any tick bites.

The Arizona case occurred on July 4th, 1973, when a 20 year old desk clerk at North Rim Lodge, Grand Canyon National Park, Arizona, developed an acute illness with headache, fever, chills and myalgia. He was discharged from hospital after four days with no diagnosis and no therapy. On July 13th, he suffered a relapse with fever (103·8°F.) and severe prostration. On readmission, spirochaetes were found in a blood smear. He recovered after tetracycline therapy.

Investigation showed that 46 of 290 employees and their family members living at the park had experienced similar illnesses during the preceding month. Sporadic cases had also occurred throughout the period June 15th to July 18th, 1973. Mouse inoculation tests on 10 patients showed all to be infected with *Borrelia sp.* The rustic cabins, where the patients resided were scattered throughout the North Rim area and included standard and de luxe cabins, dormitories for men and women employees, and the ranger housing area.

Endemic tick-borne relapsing fever has been recorded previously in Arizona and other western states, and large outbreaks can sometimes occur. The disease is transmitted by several ticks of the genus *Ornithodoros* and caused by spirochaetes of the genus *Borrelia*. The ticks hide in crevices, particularly in wood, such as is used to build log cabins, and they emerge at night to feed. Their bites often go unnoticed, because they feed in the dark for brief periods only, and the bite is relatively painless.

Rat-Bite Fever

To complete our survey of bacterial diseases, brief mention may be made of two cases of Rat-Bite Fever, reported in "Morbidity and Mortality" 23:42 (October 19th, 1974). These both occurred in technicians as a result of being bitten by laboratory rats. Cultures of *Streptobacillus moniliformis* were obtained from both patients.

Fungal Diseases

Of fungal diseases, one case reported in "Morbidity and Mortality" 22:15 (April 14th, 1973) merits attention. The condition was histoplasmosis contracted in a bat cave. On February 10th, 1973, a normally healthy 18 year old girl was admitted to hospital with severe respiratory distress; she was presumed to be suffering from influenzal pneumonia and appropriate treatment was given. However, on the third day the girl's mother reported that several of the girl's friends were suffering from a similar disease following a visit to a bat cave. Subsequently, *Histoplasma capsulatum* was cultured from a bone marrow aspirate.

Between January 1st and 21st, the patient and 28 members of a church sponsored youth group, 21 boys and 8 girls, had explored a bat infested limestone cave in Suwannee County, Florida. They entered on some two occasions and stayed in it for about 30 minutes. Attempting to encourage the bats to fly, some of the boys had thrown soil from the cave floor at them. The dusty atmosphere had induced shortness of breath in some of the explorers, who then left. Twenty-three of the party of twenty-nine were subsequently found to be infected, an attack rate of 79%. Predominant symptoms were cough, fever, night sweats, dyspnoea on exertion, malaise and chest congestion. Illness became evident 6-44 days after exposure. Histoplasma infection was confirmed by serological tests; chest x — rays showed diffuse miliary infiltrate typical of acute pulmonary histoplasmosis in 14 of 17 sick persons and in one who was clinically fit.

Histoplasmosis is most prevalent in the Mississippi and Missouri valleys. It is acquired by contact with soil containing an accumulation of bat or bird excreta. Bat habitats are often contaminated. There were only two previous reports from Florida, both associated with exploration of bat caves. It is perhaps fortunate that the bats in the cave were not carrying rabies also.

Psittacosis

Psittacosis is, of course, common in the United States associated mostly, as elsewhere, with keeping psittacine birds. A case of turkey-associated psittacosis is reported in "Morbidity and Mortality" 23:36 (September 7th, 1974). Between May 6th and June 24th, 1974, there occurred 154 cases of psittacosis among 560 employees of four turkey processing plants in Texas. Subsequently, smaller outbreaks were reported from two additional plants also in Texas, involving another 111 persons. The symptoms were fever, headache, weakness, chills and weight loss. The highest incidence occurred in the "kill and pick" departments. The turkeys implicated were from the east central area of Texas. Tests were made on 152 turkey flocks with 1 124 890 birds. Fourteen flocks from seven counties gave serological evidence of infection with *Chlamydia psittaci*. The infected flocks were quarantined and treated with chlortetracycline medicated food for 21 days before being slaughtered, since when there were no further human cases.

Viral Diseases

Rabies

We turn now to diseases caused by viruses, of which the most important zoonosis, certainly the most dreaded, is rabies. A survey of the situation in the United States for January and February 1973 is given in "Morbidity and Mortality" 22:22 (June 2nd, 1973). During these months, 494 cases of rabies in animals were reported, 104 fewer than for 1972. Of these, 366 cases (75%) were in wildlife, and of these 93% in skunks and foxes. Cases in skunks were 211 from 33 states; in foxes 131 from 13 states. Of the rest, there were 13 cases in raccoons, five in bats, four in mongoose, one each in coyote, coati mundi, and flying squirrel. In domestic animals, there were 128 cases, 78 in cattle, 27 in dogs, 13 in cats, seven in horses and mules, two in pigs and one in a sheep.

Three cases of human rabies are reported in full, all of which are worth reproducing here. The first is recorded in "Morbidity and Mortality" 22:39 (September 29th, 1973). On September 7th, 1973, a 26 year old man in Kentucky developed bilateral paraesthesia and pain in his ears, headache, sore throat and anorexia. These symptoms were later accompanied by fever, difficulty in swallowing, confusion and tremor. He was admitted to hospital with a temperature of 105°F., where the symptoms noted were nuchal rigidity, confusion, agitation and spasmodic tremors. Rabies was diagnosed serologically and by isolation of virus. In spite of heroic efforts at treatment, the patient died. He had been bitten in the ear by a bat in mid-August; the bat had escaped. Endemic wildlife rabies is known to exist in the part of Kentucky where this occurred, and bats also are infected there. The last human case occurred in 1961, when an elderly farmer died after being bitten by a fox.

The next case is reported in "Morbidity and Mortality" 22:32 (August 11th, 1973). In late June, a young skunk was found by a family in Gibson County, Tennessee, and adopted as a family pet. The family travelled to Florida a few days later and took the skunk with them. During the trip the skunk became ill and died of rabies on July 17th, after the family had returned to Tennessee. All the family were given anti-rabic treatment, and escaped infection.

Two cases of rabies exposure are reported in "Morbidity and

Mortality" 22:25 (June 23rd, 1973). In the first week of 1973, five raccoon kittens 5-6 weeks old, were found on a farm in Nashville, Kansas. Three of the raccoons died within two weeks, none of which were examined professionally. During the last week of May, the fourth raccoon was exhibited at a class at the local school and handled by many of the children. Shortly after the raccoon refused to eat, and the family attempted to force feed it by dipping their fingers in milk and placing them in the raccoon's mouth. On June 6th, the raccoon died and was found to be infected with rabies. The fifth raccoon was killed on June 6th, and was rabies negative. This episode required anti-rabic treatment, of 5 persons.

The second case occurred on May 20th, 1973. A Santa Fé College biologist trapped a wild bobcat near Gainesville, Florida. Later that day, one biologist was bitten by the animal and another was scratched. On June 1st, the bobcat was ill, and one of the biologists attempted to tube feed it. The bobcat regurgitated the food back through the tube into the biologist's face and mouth. Later that day the bobcat suffered a respiratory arrest, and mouth to mouth resuscitation was performed. The bobcat died and was found infected with rabies. Fourteen persons received anti-rabic treatment. The biologists undeservedly survived.

Equine Encephalitis

Of the arboviruses, three reports are given relating to the situation in regard to Venezuelan Equine Encephalitis in South American countries, and there is a report of an outbreak of Eastern Equine Encephalitis in "Morbidity and Mortality" 22:39 (September 29th, 1973). The latter is worth quoting. On August 1st, 1973, deaths were reported on a pheasant farm in New Hampshire. The birds suffered from a staggering gait, progressive stupor and died within a day. Horses within a 215 mile radius became sick with encephalitis and 23 died. EEE was confirmed in two horses. Following exceptionally heavy rains, there had been a great increase in numbers of *Aedes vexans* mosquitos. There were no human cases.

On August 9th, 1973, in Michigan, ten horses became ill with encephalitis and nine died. EEE was confirmed. In this case too, there had been an increase of mosquito populations. Although no human cases were reported, there had been an increase at this time of undiagnosed primary encephalitis.

Lymphocytic Choriomeningitis

A viral disease, which may be contracted from rodents is Lymphocytic Choriomeningitis (LCM). The main source of infection in the United States in recent times has been pet hamsters. The general situation was reported in "Morbidity and Mortality" 23:14 (April 6th, 1974) for the period since December 1973. Hamster contact had resulted in the occurrence of 51 cases of LCM during the five month period. There were five in California, eight in Florida, five in Massachusetts, one in Nevada, two in New Jersey and 30 in New York. All these infections came through one supplier and the source was traced. Some case histories are described in "Morbidity and Mortality" 23:8 (February 23rd, 1974):

Case 1. In late January 1974, a 24 year old woman from Rochester was admitted to hospital suffering from fever, headache, ataxia, dysarthria and urinary retention due to an atonic bladder; the illness was diagnosed as aseptic meningitis. Investigation revealed that the patient's three brothers and a close girl friend had suffered from a biphasic illness in January with headache, myalgia and fever (temperature up to 102°F.). All five persons were found to have evidence of recent LCM infection. The two other family members were negative. The family had acquired two hamsters around December 28th. The hamsters had all remained healthy, and one had delivered a litter in late January. They were all LCM positive.

Case 2. One week later, a 35 year old woman from Rochester also suffered from fever, headache and myalgia. She was found to have aseptic meningitis and was serologically positive for LCM. One of the patient's four daughters and her mother, who lived with them, had a similar illness. This family too had bought a hamster from the same source, which was LCM positive.

Three other LCM infections occurred in the same area as a result of hamster transmission. LCM is a viral disease transmissible to man by excreta or airborne infection usually from mice, but also from hamsters and guinea pigs. The clinical disease is often biphasic. The first phase is flu-like. It is followed in one or two weeks by a recurrence or the onset of meningitis or encephalomyelitis, with fever, myalgia, headache and cough. The course is usually short and rarely fatal; even when the symptoms are severe, the chances of recovery are good.

Lassa Fever

My final extract relating to viral diseases is of an investigation into "Lassa Fever", which was conducted in Sierra Leone, "Morbidity and Mortality" 22:24 (June 16th, 1973). This disease is one, which has come into prominence in recent years, because of its high mortality and for fear that it might be introduced outside Africa. In September and October 1972, epidemiological investigations were conducted in the Panguma-Tongo area in the Eastern Province of Sierra Leone. Most cases occurred during the rainy season. The overall attack rate was 2·2 per thousand; amongst patients in hospital, the death rate was 38%. Serological tests detected antibody in 13·1% of persons living in households where cases had occurred; 6·3% of persons in other households.

A total of 615 small vertebrates (480 rodents, 110 bats, 23 insectivores and two reptiles) was collected in Panguma and Tongo. Infection was found only in the multi-mammate mouse, *Mastomys natalensis.* This creature was trapped inside houses, in gardens, and in forest surrounding the villages. The isolation rate in Panguma was one in twenty six, in Tongo nine in twenty. Eight of ten isolates in Tongo were from *M. natalensis* trapped in two households inhabited by Lassa Fever patients.

Rickettsioses

Rocky Mountain Spotted Fever

It is necessary now to turn to Rocky Mountain Spotted Fever. The situation in 1972 was reviewed in "Morbidity and Mortality" 22:22 (June 2nd, 1973). In this year, there were 528 cases of RMSF, of which reliable clinical reports were available from 212. Of these cases, 95% were from five states, Alabama, North Carolina, Ohio, Tennessee and Virginia. The Rocky Mountain states reported fewer cases. Children under 19 years old accounted for 151 (71%) of the cases. Eleven patients died. The following case histories are quoted from "Morbidity and Mortality" 23:35 (August 31st, 1974): —

Case 1. On May 29th, 1974, an eight year old boy from central Louisiana developed fever, malaise and lassitude. Next day, a rash developed on both wrists and spread to his face, trunk and extremities. A preliminary diagnosis was made of varicella, but was changed the next day to scarlatina, for which oral penicillin was given. On June 5th, seven days after onset, the temperature was 105°F. and there was lethargy and personality changes. He was then admitted to hospital, and found to have a generalised petechial exanthem involving his face, neck, trunk, upper and lower extremities, and the palms and soles of his feet. There were bilateral conjunctival petechiae, injected throat, and systemic lymphadenopathy. The parents then revealed that the boy had suffered numerous tick bites, and a tick had indeed been removed the day before onset. A diagnosis was then made of Rocky Mountain Spotted Fever and tetracycline therapy was started some five hours after admission to hospital. Over the next three days, the boy developed gastrointestinal haemorrhage, cardio-respiratory arrest, aspiration pneumonia and progressive neurological deterioration. By June 8th, respirations and reflexes were absent, and the pupils were dilated and fixed. After 24 hours maintenance by respirator, he was pronounced dead.

Case 2. On May 12th, a 61 year old man, from whom a tick had been removed on May 8th, developed malaise and generalised aches. Over the next five days, he had headache, conjunctivitis, photophobia and fever. On May 20th, he was found unconscious with seizures and was sent to hospital. Rocky Mountain Spotted Fever was suspected and he was treated with tetracycline and other drugs. After two days, he was transferred to another hospital, comatose and with a generalised petechial rash. Over the next week he developed neurological symptoms, and the clinical course was complicated by renal failure, which required haemo-dialysis. He died on June 11th as a result of progressive cerebral impairment.

Case 3. On May 19th, 1974, a 12 year old boy from Richmond, Virgina, became ill with a temperature of 103°F. Tick bites were noted and there was posterior occipital lymphadenopathy associated with pharyngitis. He was treated with aspirin, but the fever continued and intermittent vomiting developed. On May 22nd, he was returned to the doctor with a temperature of 100°F. and a morbilliform rash on the face and chest. On May 25th the patient was still vomiting, and he was given anti-nausea suppositories. On May 28th, he became stuporous and unstable on his feet; he had two convulsions. He was taken to hospital and received phenobarbital sedation; treatment was begun with chloramphenicol. However, he died within 24 hours. The boys' serum on May 27th, was strongly positive for RMSF.

Typhus

The early diagnosis of RMSF presents difficulty, and other febrile exanthemata are often suspected. It is to be supposed that all the cases quoted above would have recovered if correct treatment had been given in time. Cases of murine typhus occasionally occur in the United States. The two accounts that follow are taken from "Morbidity and Mortality" 22:43 (November 2nd, 1973): —

Case 1. An 11 year old girl from Lincoln, Nebraska, developed an illness with fever, headache, stupor, malaise, myalgia, splenomegaly and a petechial rash on May 17th, 1973. On admission to hospital on

May 23rd, the rash was noted to involve the palms and soles of the feet. The child had received a tick bite on May 10th, and serological tests indicated infection with a typhus group fever. The presumptive diagnosis was Rocky Mountain Spotted Fever. Investigation revealed that from April 22nd to 28th, 1973, the patient had accompanied her stepfather to McAllen, Texas, an area endemic for murine typhus. The incubation period of 8 to 12 days was unusually long for murine typhus, but it was thought that the child's dog could have picked up infected fleas and acted as a transient carrier. Fleas from cats have been implicated in transmitting murine typhus, so that this supposition is not far-fetched.

Case 2. A 51 year old man from Edgemont, South Dakota, was admitted to hospital on May 30th, 1973. He complained of fever and a generalised rash of one day's duration. The patient had had a flu-like prodrome for the previous ten days. On admission, he had a generalised maculo-papular rash, dark red in colour, and a temperature of 105°F. The presumptive diagnosis was Rocky Mountain Spotted Fever. The symptoms subsided on antibiotic treatment in seven days. Serological tests showed a typhus type fever. This patient had not left the area of his home, where typhus fevers would not be expected. However, the serological picture was compatible with recrudescent epidemic typhus (Brill-Zinsser Disease). The patient reported having had a febrile illness compatible with typhus in Liège, Belgium, during his military service with the US army in 1944.

Scrub Typhus (Tsutsugamushi Disease)

Two further rickettsioses are reported from the United States, acquired in foreign parts, which must have caused their diagnosticians some difficulty and are worth recounting. The first of these was a case of Scrub Typhus or Tsutsugamushi Disease acquired in Japan, described in "Morbidity and Mortality" 23:11 (March 16th, 1974):

On November 25th, 1973, a 38 year old man from Greenwich, Connecticut, developed an acute illness with fever, headache and maculo-papular rash after returning from a vacation in Japan. At first, he was thought to have systemic generalised vaccinia, following vaccination on November 6th. In spite of vaccinia immune globulin, his illness progressed with splenomegaly, right lower lobe pneumonitis and symptoms of encephalitis. There was no lymphadenopathy. The patient had taken a trip to the Mount Fujiyama region, the base of which is an endemic scrub typhus area. He had walked through low scrub, where he could have been bitten by an infected mite. Three days later, an eschar had developed on his left ankle. The patient recovered with tetracycline treatment. Tsutsugamushi is primarily a rural or sylvan disease, where ecological "mite islands" as small as 1 m² may serve as reservoirs and intense foci of infection. The untreated disease is frequently severe and often fatal, but prompt diagnosis and treatment with tetracycline or chloramphenicol usually results in complete recovery.

African Tick Typhus

A case of African Tick Typhus is described in "Morbidity and Mortality" 22:42 (October 20th, 1973). On June 16th, 1973, a 53 year old woman on Rhode Island became ill with an influenza-like condition with fever (101°F.), malaise, myalgia, headache and rhinitis. She also had 13 painful skin lesions on her forearms, thighs and popliteal areas, which were erythematous and raised with a pustular centre. There was no cough or conjunctivitis, and no adenopathy. Between June 1st and 13th the patient had visited friends in Kloof, Natal, South Africa. After her return to USA, a telegram was received to say that her hostess had contracted Tick Typhus. Though she had no memory of a tick bite, she had spent a day riding in a jeep in a game reserve and she had been in her hostess' garden. Serological findings were consistent with African Tick Fever infection.

Protozoal Diseases

Giardiasis

Without constant vigilance, the rickettsioses could plainly pose a serious problem in a country so large and diverse as the United States. Protozoal diseases present a lesser problems, except for malaria. There are constant references in the reports to malaria, either outbreaks in contiguous countries or cases which have occurred in malaria free areas. These do not concern us, and we may mention briefly two protozoal zoonoses, which are of interest but little practical importance. The first of these is giardiasis, caused by a flagellate, *Giardia lamblia.* The first report is in "Morbidity and Mortality" 23:50 (December 14th, 1974): —

In Utah, 34 of 52 campers developed gastrointestinal symptoms compatible with giardiasis and stool samples confirmed infection with *G. lamblia.* They had drunk water from a mountain stream, the infection evidently came from wildlife contamination of the water, most likely beavers though domestic sheep possibly could have been the source. The second report is in "Morbidity and Mortality" 23:9 (March 2nd, 1974), and appeared in travellers returned from the

Soviet Union. A party of 399 nurses visited Leningrad and Moscow in May 1973. Of those, from whom stool specimens were obtained, 43% were positive for *G. lamblia.* A few were asymptomatic, the rest suffered symptoms of varying severity. It is not uncommon to contract giardiasis in the Soviet Union, which apparently results from drinking untreated tap water. The main symptoms are diarrhoea, the stools being often greasy and malodorous, abdominal cramps, fatigue, weight loss, flatulence, anorexia and nausea. Records show that in other travellers 23% of 1419 have suffered infection.

Babesiosis

A case of babesiosis is reported in "Morbidity and Mortality" 22:39 (September 29th, 1973). On September 4th, 1973, a 48 year old woman living on Nantucket Island, Massachusetts, complained of daily recurrent chills, fever and myalgia in her legs and side, that had begun one week before. She had moderately severe depression, but no diarrhoea, rash, adenopathy, or splenomegaly. She had suffered a tick bite in mid-August; this became inflamed and a local abscess containing the tick head was excised. Rocky Mountain Spotted Fever was suspected, but there was no response to tetracycline therapy. Meanwhile, the temperature rose to 104°F. and blood smears were found to be positive for *Babesia microti.* The condition was cured by chloroquine. The source of the tick is uncertain. The patient had two dogs, but no other pets or farm animals. However, this babesia is not a parasite of dogs, but may have been harboured by rats which lived under the house. Babesiosis is very rare in the United States, and only two other cases have been reported one of them probably acquired on Nantucket Island. This excludes cases in persons, who have had their spleens removed, which suggests that the scarcity of infection is more a matter of resistance to it than absence of babesia parasites.

Helminth Infections

Canine Heartworm

Reports of helminth infections are also somewhat scanty, except for trichinosis, which is important and serious. First, we shall quote a single report of infection with the dog heartworm—"Morbidity and Mortality" 23:44 (November 2nd, 1974). The heartworm, *Dirofilaria immitis* is a serious parasite of dogs in some of the southern states. In parts of Louisiana it is so widespread that almost all dogs contract it sooner or later. The adult worms live in the chambers of the heart causing cardiac symptoms and irreversible liver changes, resulting in death. Treatment is unsatisfactory and often of itself fatal. The worms are transmitted by mosquitoes, which acquire the microfilariae during the course of a blood meal. The human case is described as under: —

A 48 year old man became affected with bilateral asymptomatic pulmonary nodules. An exploratory operation revealed nodules of *Dirofilaria immitis*. The patient was born and raised in Sitka, Alaska, but had lived in southern New Mexico and south California. He went to Houston to work as a labourer and was often bitten by mosquitos. Where he contracted the infection is not clear. The first case of human heartworm infection was reported in 1961, since when there have been 21 cases. The symptoms are cough and chest pain, sometimes haemoptysis, malaise, myalgia, chills and fever. Half the cases are asymptomatic. Differential diagnosis is difficult. Though radiography is helpful, surgery is necessary. Usually a single worm is found located in a medium sized artery, surrounded by a zone of infarction. The worms never develop to maturity in man and microfilariae are never found.

Trichinosis

Trichinosis is an ever present threat in the United States. The position in 1972 was surveyed in "Morbidity and Mortality" 22:46 (November 17th, 1973). During this year, 96 cases of trichinosis were reported, the severity being mild to severe with one death. There were eight outbreaks involving at least two cases; one involved four persons and seven cases involved two to three persons. The majority of cases are acquired from eating commercially prepared pork products consumed at home. Of the fifty states, 11 reported at least one case, but 66% were from New York, New Jersey, Illinois, and California. All three individual cases reported are worthy of quotation. The first is found in "Morbidity and Mortality" 22:34 (August 25th, 1973): —

On March 11th, 1973, a 30 year old woman in Perry County, Ohio, became ill with fever, chills, malaise and periorbital oedema. She was admitted to hospital three days later. Her blood showed 8% eosinophilia and her serum was positive for trichinosis. Biopsy revealed severe muscle necrosis and phagocytosis with inflammatory myopathy. Non-encysted larvae of *Trichinella spiralis* were also present. She died in hospital on April 15th. About March 18th, the patient's 13 year old son developed symptoms compatible with mild trichinosis. On admission to hospital, his serum was found positive for *T. spiralis*. The patient and her son had on several occasions between February 10th and March 18th, eaten pork chops, which had been cooked for a short time. Some chops remained in the freezer and were found to be infected with *T. spiralis*. The next report comes from "Morbidity and Mortality" 22:36 (September 8th, 1973): —

On June 27th, 1973, a 29 year old man was admitted to hospital with symptoms compatible with a cerebrovascular accident, that is "stroke". The history included fever, periorbital oedema and weakness of the left side, but no associated headaches, visual symptoms or sensory disturbances. There were weaknesses in certain muscles, and left hemiparesis with greater involvement of the lower than the upper extremity. He was unable to move his toes. A blood count revealed 52% eosinophilia of 11 200 white cells, and the serum was positive for trichinosis. He responded satisfactorily to treatment with thiabendazole, prednisone and a tranquillizer. At the time of discharge, the patient had mild weakness of the left upper extremity and the left lower extremity, but could walk without assistance. The diagnosis was a cerebrovascular accident secondary to angiitis with a hypersensitive reaction to *T. spiralis* infection. The man was in the habit of eating raw hamburgers from several markets in Baltimore County. Adulterated ground beef was the suspected vehicle. The third case is taken from "Morbidity and Mortality" 22:23 (June 9th, 1973): —

Between January 14th and 29th, 1973, 15 of 25 members of four families became ill with fever (93%), diarrhoea (73%), muscle aches (67%), periorbital oedema (53%) and headache (47%). Three were admitted to hospital, one with pneumonia and severe muscle aches, one with nephritis, and one with evidence of myocarditis and involvement of the central nervous system. Trichinosis was diagnosed serologically; treatment was successful and none died. Of the other four family members, three children were found affected but asymptomatic.

On December 26th, Family 1 had butchered two brood sows and one beef animal; two days later sausages were made. The sausage mince was packed in natural casing, not smoked, and hung dry until January 6th, 1973, when it was divided between families 1 and 2. On January 7th, family 2 gave a card party, at which families 3 and 4 were present; the sausage was served uncooked. Five members of the three families became ill. Samples of the remaining sausage and of pork chops from the same source were infected with *T. spiralis*. The source of infection in the sows remains obscure. The pig herd was managed on a closed system, and none of some 330 other pigs was found infected. Rats on the farm were also found to be free from infection. Nevertheless, there must have been some wildlife source.

Marine Zoonoses

To end this review we turn back to marine life. We have already seen how marine animals can concentrate and transmit enteric organisms and the virus of infectious hepatitis. We have also seen how they can harbour a pathogenic marine-living organism, *Vibrio parahaemolyticus*. Our sources give an account of three cases of shellfish poisoning associated with "red tides" all of which are worth quoting, and one of "ciguatera" in Hawaii. The first report is found in "Morbidity and Mortality" 22:48 (December 1st, 1973): —

On November 17th, 1973, a two year old boy experienced circumoral paraesthesias, intermittent diplopia, dizziness, thirst, fatigue, nausea and vomiting 30 minutes after eating steamed clams, gathered on a beach in Sarasota County, Florida. His 10 year old companion ate five clams and also became ill within 30 minutes with similar symptoms, and later experienced dysphonia, ataxia and weakness of the legs. Some four hours after eating the clams, he had a generalised convulsion and was admitted to a local hospital. Following a respiratory arrest he was unresponsive with dilated pupils and paralysis. Over the next four days he recovered completely.

On November 18th, shortly after consuming 3-4 dozen steamed clams from a beach in Sarasota Bay, a man and woman developed paraesthesia in their mouths and later of the extremities, nausea, vomiting and fatigue. The next morning, they had persistent weakness and paraesthesias of their extremities; in addition, the man developed abdominal pain and diarrhoea. Both recovered.

The area, where these clams were collected, had been closed to commercial exploitation for some years because of pollution, so that the clams were not distributed widely. Elevated numbers of the dinoflagellate, *Gymnodinium breve*, had been detected in the area in October and a red tide alert had been declared. There had also been a small fish kill, but no bird deaths were reported. Residents of many coastal areas in Sarasota County had experienced symptoms of conjunctival and upper respiratory tract irritation. Clams from the area were found, on testing in mice, to be high in *G. breve* toxin.

G. breve is responsible for the red tides along the Florida Coast. *Gonyaulax tamarensis* cause them along the north eastern coast of the United States. *Gonyaulax catanella* is responsible for most red tides along the Pacific coast. With the exception of the convulsion, the symptoms and signs were typical of red tide-associated shellfish poisoning. Symptoms were more severe than usual with *G. breve*, but less severe than those from gonyaulax toxin. The next report comes from "Morbidity and Mortality" 23:12 (March 23rd, 1974): —

At midnight on March 10th, 1974, a 20 year old man from Englewood, Florida, began experiencing an unusual sensation around his face and mouth, which he described as "plastic". At 4.00 a.m., he woke with abdominal cramps, severe leg cramps, tight leg muscles and a burning facial sensation. At 6.30 a.m., he was taken to the emergency ward of a hospital, where he appeared oriented but agitated. He had no fever, but the heart rate was 130/minute, blood pressure 14/100 and respiratory rate 20/minute. He appeared to respond to symptomatic treatment and returned home. Three hours later, he had leg cramps more severe than before, cramps in his arms and chest, a suffocating feeling, abnormal posturing and numbness of the hands and feet. He was admitted to hospital and discharged on March 12th.

Three hours before becoming ill, he and two friends had eaten clams that they had dug earlier in the day. The clams came from the beach along the bay near Englewood, where a red tide caused by *Gymnodinium breve* had been reported. Some of the clams had been steamed in beer for 30-40 minutes and some had been baked and fried. The patient ate about two dozen cooked clams, a companion ate ten cooked clams, and the other ate one raw clam. All three drank a large quantity of beer and smoked marijuana after the meal. Neither of the two companions became ill. Clams reclaimed from the refrigerator and collected from the beach contained large amounts of toxin. The final episode is taken from "Morbidity and Mortality" 23:37 (September 14th, 1974): —

On August 31st, 1974, a 38 year old woman experienced pectoral paraesthesias 15 minutes after eating two dozen steamed mussels, which she had gathered earlier that day from Rye Beach, New Hampshire. Within four hours, she developed generalised weakness, dysphonia and vomiting. She was admitted to hospital, where she had a respiratory arrest from which she was resuscitated. As from September 9th, she had recovered except for some residual paraesthesias. Three other persons were affected, but less severely, and recovered. The mussels were examined and contained high levels of a neurotoxin also present in the vomit of the patients. This was associated with unusually high numbers of *Gonyaulax tamarensis* in the coastal waters; the beaches had been closed to shellfish harvesting before the mussels were collected. To end this review, we will discuss the sole report of "ciguatera", "Morbidity and Mortality" 23:23 (June 8th, 1974): —

In February and early March 1974, a number of cases of neurological illnesses were reported in Hawaii, which suggested the disease of ciguatera resulting from the consumption of "kahala" (amberjack or *Seriola drumerilii*) fish weighing 30 lbs or more. On the afternoon of March 10th a physician reported to the local health department that he had seen a number of patients with diarrhoea, weakness, paraesthesias and paradoxical temperature sensation. All sick persons had eaten small amounts of kahala sashimi — raw, spiced amberjack — at a restaurant, which had served groups at about 7.30 p.m. on March 9th. One of the groups, a wedding party of 110 persons, was investigated. Of them, 57 were interviewed and 29 (51%) had been ill with diarrhoea or neurological symptoms. The mean incubation period was 12 hours. The fish produced illness in mongoose compatible with ciguatera. A second group, who ate the fish, also had symptoms but the mean incubation period was seven hours; they ate the fish in chunks, kahala nitsuke.

The two amberjacks served at the restaurant had been caught on March 3rd and frozen until the day of the outbreak; one weighed 20 lb and the other 30 lb. The fish were cleaned at noon by the chef on March 9th. Viscera from the 30 lb fish were sautéed in soy sauce and eaten that afternoon by the chef. He immediately had symptoms in the mouth of tingling and within 1½ hours he developed abdominal cramps, diarrhoea and paraesthesia of his extremities.

Ciguatera is a form of ichthyosarcotoxicosis caused by ingestion of marine shore or reef fish in tropical or sub-tropical waters. Over 400 species of fish are reported to be ciguatoxic, but the barracuda is the commonest to cause outbreaks; others are amberjack, red snapper and grouper. The toxin is heat stable, not toxic to the fish, and concentrated mostly in the liver, intestinal tract, testes, ovaries and muscles. Large fish are more likely to be toxic than small. The toxin is believed to be derived from marine protozoa.

Bibliography

Ahuja, L. (1958). Rabies in India. *J. trop. Med. Hyg.* **61,** 95-99.

Allmond, B. W. jr., Froeschle, J. E. and Guilloud, N. D. (1967). Paralytic poliomyelitis in large laboratory primates; virological investigation and report on the use of oral poliomyelitis virus (OPV) vaccine. *Am. J. Epidem.* **85,** 229-239.

Amelsfoort, V. F. P. M. van (1964). "Culture, Stone Age and Modern Medicine." Assen (Netherlands): van Gorcum.

Andrewes, Sir C. (1964). "Viruses of Vertebrates." London: Bailliére, Tindall and Cox.

Bach, F. W., Fuelscher, J. and Harnack, . (1931). Ueber eine durch Affen verursachte Ruhrepidemie. *Veroeff. Med. Verw.* **00,** 61-73.

Banks, A. L. (1969). Catastrophe and restraints. *In* "Population and Food Supply." (Hutchinson, Sir J.) Cambridge: Cambridge University Press.

Beautyman, W. and Woolf, A. L. (1951).
J. Path. Bact. **63,** 635.

Beverley, J. K. A. (1974). Some aspects of toxoplasmosis, a world-wide zoonosis. *In* "Parasitic Zoonoses." (Soulsby, E. J. L., ed.). London: Academic Press.

Beveridge, W. I. B. (1977). "Influenza: the Last Great Plague." London: Heinemann.

Bibby, G. (1962a). "The Testimony of the Spade. Life in Northern Europe from 15 000 BC to the Time of the Vikings." London: Collins (Fontana).

Bibby, G. (1962b). "Four Thousand Years Ago: a Panorama of Life in the Second Century BC." London: Collins.

Bisseru, B. (1967). "Diseases of Man acquired from his Pets." London: Heinemann.

Black, F. L. (1966).
J. theoret. Biol. **11,** 207.

Boulger, L. (1966). Natural rabies in a laboratory monkey. *Lancet* **00,** 941-943.

Bourlière, F. (1959). Lifespans of wild animals. *In* "The Lifespan of Animals." pp. 91-92. CIBA Foundation Symposium.

Bourne, A. (1972). "Pollute and be Damned." London: J. M. Dent.

Bourne, A. (1975). "The Man/Food Equation." *In* Steele, E. and Bourne, A. (eds). London: Academic Press.

Bourne, A. (1976). The ecological basis of the urban situation. *In* "Environment of Human Settlements." (Lacoste, P.). Oxford: Pergamon.

Bray, R. S. (1974). Zoonoses in leishmaniasis. *In* "Parasitic Zoonoses." (Soulsby, E. J. L., ed.). London: Academic Press.

Burnet, Sir M. (1960). "Principles of Animal Virology." London: Academic Press.

Burnet, Sir M. (1962). "Natural History of Infectious Diseases." Cambridge: Cambridge University Press.

Burton, J. D. and Leatherhead, T. M. (1971). Mercury in a coastal marine environment. *Nature* **231,** 440-441.

Carpenter, K. P. and Sandiford, B. R. (1952). Epidemiology of a human case of bacillary dysentery due to infection by *Shigella flexneri* 103Z. *Br. Med. J.* **i,** 142-143.

Cockburn, A. (1963). "The Evolution and Eradication of Infectious Diseases." Baltimore: Johns Hopkins Press.

Cole, S. (1965). "The Neolithic Revolution." London: British Museum (Natural History).

Cornwall, I. W. (1959). Geochronology. *In* "Chambers Encyclopaedia". London: Newnes.

Deevey, E. J. jr. (1971). The human population. *In* "Man and the Ecosphere." (Ehrlich, P. R., Holdren, J. P. and Holm, R. W., eds). San Francisco: Freeman and Co.

Dempster, J. P. (1975). "Animal Population Ecology." London: Academic Press.

Doory, Y. al (1972). Superficial, intermediate and systemic mycoses. *In* "Pathology of Simian Primates." (Fiennes, R. N. T-W-). Basel: Karger.

Dudgeon, L. S. and Urquhart, A. L. (1919). A system of bacteriology. *Spec. Rep. Ser. Med. Res. Comm. London.*

Eckholm, E. P. (1976). "Losing Ground." N.Y.: Norton.

Ehrlich, P. R. and Ehrlich, A. H. (1970). "Population, Resources, Environment." San Francisco: Freeman.

Ehrlich, P. R., Ehrlich, A. H. and Holdren, J. P. (1973). "Human Ecology." San Francisco: Freeman.

Felsenfeld, A. D. (1972). The arboviruses. *In* "Pathology of Simian Primates." Part II. (Fiennes, R. N. T-W-, ed.). pp. 523-534. Basel; Karger.

Fenner, F. (1971). Infectious disease and social change. *Med. J. of Australia*, May 15th **1**, 1043 and May 22nd **1**, 1099.

Fiennes, R. N. T-W- (1940). "A note on a dysentery-like organism isolated from the intestinal contents of a calf." *E.A. Med. J.* **7**, 122-124.

Fiennes, R. N. T-W- (1964). "Man, Nature and Disease." London: Weidenfeld and Nicolson, N.Y.: Signet Science Series.

Fiennes, R. N. T-W- (1967). "Zoonoses of Primates." London: Weidenfeld and Nicolson, Cornell: Cornell University Press.

Fiennes, R. N. T-W- (1972) (ed.). (1972). "Pathology of Simian Primates." Basel: Karger.

Fiennes, R. N. T-W- (1972). Rabies. *In* "Pathology of Simian Primates." Part II. (Fiennes, R. N. T-W-). pp. 646-661. Basel: Karger.

Fiennes, R. N. T-W- (1972). Ectoparasites and vectors. *In* "Pathology of Simian Primates." (Fiennes, R. N. T-W-, ed.). pp. 158-173. Basel: Karger.

Fiennes, R. N. T-W- (1972). Tuberculosis of primates. *In* "Pathology of Simian Primates." Part II (Fiennes, R. N. T-W-, ed.). pp. 314-333. Basel: Karger.

Fiennes, R. N. T-W-, Pinkerton, M. and Dzhikidze, K. (1972). Enteropathogenic organisms. *In* "Pathology of Simian Primates." Part II (Fiennes, R. N. T-W-, ed.). pp. 277-281. Basel: Karger.

Findlay, C. M., MacCallum, F. O. and Murgatroyd, F. (1939). Observations on the aetiology of infective hepatitis (so-called epidemic catarrhal jaundice). *T. R. Soc. Med. Hyg.* **32**, 575.

Fribourg-Blanc, A. (1972). Treponema. *In* "Pathology of Simian Primates." (Fiennes, R. N. T-W-, ed.). pp. 255-261. Basel: Karger.

Garnham, P. C. C. (1966). "Malaria Parasites and other Haemosporidia." Oxford: Blackwell.

Gross, L. (1970). "Oncogenic Viruses." 2nd edition. Oxford: Pergamon.

Hackett, C. J. (1975). An introduction to diagnostic criteria of syphilis, treponarid and yaws (treponematoses) in dry bones and some implications. *Virchow's Arch. A. Path. Anat. and Histol.* **368**, 229-241.

Heberling, R. L. (1972). The Simian picornaviruses. *In* "Pathology of Simian Primates." Part II (Fiennes, R. N. T-W-, ed.). pp. 497-512. Basel: Karger.

Hicks, Sir C. S. (1975). "Man and Natural Resources." London: Croom Helm.

Hoeden, J. van der (1964). "Zoonoses." Amsterdam: Elsevier.

Hollingsworth, T. H. (1973). Population crises in the past. *In* "Population and the New Biology." (Benjamin, B., Cox, P. R. and Peel, J., eds). London: Academic Press.

Holmes, A. W., Wolfe, L. and Deinhardt, F. (1972). Infectious hepatitis in marmosets. *In* "Pathology of Simian Primates." Part II (Fiennes, R. N. T-W-, ed.). pp. 684-700. Basel: Karger.

Hurst, W. W. and Pawan, J. L. (1931). A further account of the Trinidad outbreak of acute rabic myelitis. *J. Path. Bact.* **35**, 301-321.

Hutner, S. H., Baker, H., Frank, O. and Cox, D. (1972). Nutrition and metabolism in protozoa. *In* "Biology of Nutrition." (Fiennes, R. N. T-W-, ed.). Oxford: Pergamon.

Innes, J. R. M. and Saunders, I. Z. (1962). "Comparative Neuropathology." N.Y. and London: Academic Press.

Iverson, J. (1971). Forest clearance in the Stone Age. *In* "Man and the Ecosphere." (Ehrlich, P. R., Holdren, J. P. and Holm, R. W., eds). San Francisco: Freeman.

Johnson, H. N. (1959). Rabies. *In* "Viral and Rickettsial Infections of Man." (Rivers, T. M. and Horsfall, F. L.). Philadelphia: Lippincott.

Johnston, R. (ed.). (1976). "Marine Pollution." London: Academic Press.

Jubb, K. V. F. and Kennedy, P. C. (1963). "Pathology of Domestic Animals". Vol. 1. N.Y. and London: Academic Press.

Kalter, S. S. (1972). Serologic surveys. *In* "Pathology of Simian Primates." Part II (Fiennes, R. N. T-W-, ed.). pp. 469-490. Basel: Karger.

Kaplan, C. (ed.). (1977). "Rabies the Facts." London: Oxford University Press.

Keymer, I. F. (1974). Ornithosis in free living and captive birds. *Proc. R. Soc. Med.* **67**, 733-735.

Kurstan, E. and Maramorosch, K. (eds) (1974). "Viruses, Evolution and Cancer." N.Y. and London: Academic Press.

Lange, W. L. (1969). The black death. *In* "Man and the Ecosphere." (Ehrlich, P. R., Holdren, J. P. and Holm, R. W., eds). San Francisco: Freeman.

Lapin, B. A. and Yakovleva, L. A. (1963). "Comparative Pathology in Monkeys." Springfield: Thomas.

Macintosh, N. W. G. (1967). Fossil Man in Australia. *Aust. J. Sci.* **30**, 86-98.

Moller-Christensen, N. V. (1961). "Bone Changes in Leprosy." Copenhagen: Munksgaard, Bristol: John Wright.

Mulligan, H. W. (ed.) (1970). "The African Trypanosomiases." London: Allen & Unwin.

Mulvaney, D. J. (1966). The prehistory of the Australian Aborigine. *Scientific American* **214**, 84-91.

Onyango, R. J., Hoeve, K. van and Raadt, P. de (1966). The epidemiology of *T. rhodesiense* sleeping sickness in Alego Location, Central Nyanza, Kenya. I. Evidence that cattle may act as reservoir hosts of trypanosomes infective to man. *T. R. Soc. trop. Med. Hyg.* **60**, 175.

Orihel, T. C. and Seibold, H. R. (1972). Nematodes of the bowel and tissues. *In* "Pathology of Simian Primates." Part I (Fiennes, R. N. T-W-, ed.). pp. 76-99. Basel: Karger.

Pollitzer, R. (1959). "Cholera." Geneva: WHO.

Probstmayer, R. (1863). "Dictionary of Veterinary Sciences."

Rabin, H. (1978). Studies in nonhuman primates with exogenous type-C and type-D oncornaviruses. *In* "Recent Advances in Primatology." Vol. 4 (Chivers, D. J. and Ford, E. H. R., eds). London: Academic Press.

Reichenbach-Klinke, H. and Elkan, E. (1965). "The Principal Diseases of Lower Vertebrates." N.Y. and London: Academic Press.

Rickets, H. T. (1906). The study of Rocky Mountain Spotted Fever by means of animal inoculation. *J. am. Med. Ass.* **47**, 30.

Ricketts, H. T. (1907). The role of the wood tick, *Dermacentor occidentalis* in Rocky Mountain Spotted Fever and the susceptibility of local animals to the disease. *J. am. med. Ass.* **49**, 24.

Ricketts, H. T. (1909). A micro-organism which apparently has a specific relationship to Rocky Mountain Spotted Fever. *J. am. med. Ass.* **52**, 379.

Shope, R. E. (1931). Swine Influenza, 1. Experimental transmission and pathology. *J. exp. Med.* **54**, 349-359.

Shope, R. E. (1936). The incidence of neutralizing antibodies for swine influenza virus in the sera of human beings of different ages. *J. exp. Med.* **63**, 669-684.

Shope, R. E. (1943). The swine lungworm as a reservoir and intermediate host for swine influenza virus. 4. The demonstration of masked swine influenza virus in lungworm larvae and swine under natural conditions. *J. exp. Med* **77**, 127-138.

Shope, R. E. (1955). The swine lungworm as a reservoir for swine influenza virus. 5. Provocation of swine influenza by exposure of prepared swine to adverse weather. *J. exp. Med.* **102**, 567-572.

Simpson, D. I. H. (1972). Other virus diseases—simian haemorrhagic fever, marburg virus, kuru and other degenerative conditions. *In* "Pathology of Simian Primates." Part II (Fiennes, R. N. T-W-, ed.). pp. 702-712, Basel: Karger.

Smetana, H. F. (1972). Infectious hepatitis. *In* "Pathology of Simian Primates." Part II (Fiennes, R. N. T-W-, ed.). pp. 663-680. Basel: Karger.

Soulsby, E. J. L. (ed.) (1974). "Parasitic Zoonoses." London: Academic Press.

Sulkin, J. E. and Allen, M. R. (1974). "Virus Infections of Bats." Basel: Karger.

Tierkel, E. S. (1964). Rabies. *In* "Zoonoses." (Hoeden, J. van der). Amsterdam, London, N.Y.: Elsevier.

UFAW (1976). "Handbook on the Care and Management of Laboratory Animals." Edinburgh, London and N.Y.: Churchill Livingstone.

"Virus Cancer Program" (1975, 1976, 1977). NIH, US Dept. of Health, Education and Welfare.

Vischer, A. L. (1947). "Old Age, Its Compensations and Rewards." London: Allen and Unwin.

Voller, A. (1972). Plasmodium and hepatocystis. *In* "Pathology of Simian Primates." Part II (Fiennes, R. N. T-W-, ed.), pp. 57-65. Basel: Karger.

Wells, C. (1964). "Bones, Bodies and Disease." London: Thames and Hudson.

Williamson, B. (1977). Unravelling the genetics of a blood disease. *New Scientist* **75**, 406-408.

Wilson, G. S. and Miles, A. A. (1953). "Topley and Wilson's Principles of Bacteriology and Immunity." 4th edition: London.

WHO (Annual Publications). "World Survey of Rabies." Geneva: WHO.

Woodruff, A. W. (1969). Epilepsy and fever in helminthic infections transmitted from animals. *Proc. R. Soc. Med.* **62**, 1045-1046.

Woodruff, A. W., Ashton, H. and Stott, G. (1961). *T. Roy. Soc. Trop. Med. Hyg.* **55**, 13.

Yanasigawa, K. (1958). "The Effect of BCG Vaccination upon Occurrence of Leprosy." Trans. 7th Int. Cong. Leprosy pp. 351-356. Tokyo: Jap. Leprosy Foundation.

Zdrovskii, P. F. and Golinevich, E. H. (1960). "The Rickettsial Diseases." Oxford: Pergamon.

Ziegler, P. (1969). "The Black Death." London: Collins.

Zinsser, H. (1935). "Rats, Lice and History." London: Routledge.

Supplementary Reference List

The references under are not quoted in the text, but have been used in compilation of the material. They are included for reasons given in the Introduction.

Influenza

Beveridge, W. I. B. (1975). The origin of influenza pandemics. *WHO Chronicle* **29,** 471-473.

Easterday, B. C., Laver, W. G., Pereira, H. G. and Schild, G. C. (1969). Antigenic composition of recombinant virus strains produced from human and avian influenza A viruses. *J. gen. Virol.* **5,** 89-91.

Kilbourne, E. D. (1968). Recombination of influenza A viruses of human and animal origin. *Science* **160,** 74.

Kilbourne, E. D., Lief, F. S. Schulman, J. L., Jahiel, R. I. and Laver, W. G. (1967). Antigenic hybrids of influenza viruses and their implications. *Perspect. Virol.* **5,** 87.

Laver, W. G. and Webster, R. G. (1972). Antibodies to human influenza virus neuraminidase (the A-Asian-57 H2N2 strain) in sera from Australian pelagic birds. *Bull. Wld Hlth Org.* **47,** 535-541.

Laver, W. G. and Webster, R. G. (1973). Studies on the origin of pandemic influenza. 3. Evidence implicating duck and equine influenza viruses as possible progenitors of the Hong Kong strain of human influenza. *Virology,* **51,** 383-391.

McCanon, D. and Schild, G. C. (1972). Segregation of antigenic and biological characteristics during influenza virus recombination. *J. gen. Virol.* **15,** 73-77.

Schild, G. C. and Newman, R. W. (1969). Immunological relationships between neuraminidases of human and animal influenza viruses. *Bull. Wld Hlth Org.* **41,** 437-445.

Tumova, B. and Schild, G. C. (1972). Antigenic relationships between type A influenza viruses of human, porcine, equine and avian origin. *Bull. Wld Hlth Org.* **47,** 453-460.

Webster, R. G. (1969). Antigenic variation in influenza viruses with special reference to Hong Kong influenza. *Bull. Wld Hlth Org.* **41,** 483-485.

Webster, R. G. (1970). Antigenic hybrids of influenza A viruses with surface antigens to order. *Virology* **42,** 633-642.

Webster, R. G. (1972). On the origin of pandemic influenza viruses. *Current Topics in Microbiology and Immunology* **59,** 75-105.

Webster, R. G. and Campbell, C. H. (1972). The *in vivo* production of a "new" influenza virus. II. *In vivo* isolation of the "new" virus. *Virology* **48,** 528-536.

Webster, R. G., Campbell, C. H. and Granoff, A. (1971). The *in vivo* production of "new" influenza A viruses. I. Genetic recombination between avian and mammalian influenza viruses. *Virology* 44, 317-328.

World Health Organization (1972). Influenza in animals. *Bull. Wld Hlth Org.* 47, 439-541.

Cancer

Baltimore, D. (1970). Viral RNA-dependent DNA polymerase in virions of RNA tumour viruses. *Nature* 226, 1209-1211.

Bittner, J. J. (1936). Some possible effects of nursing on the mammary gland tumour incidence in mice. *Science* 84, 162.

Ellerman, V. and Bang, O. (1908). Experimentelle leukamie bei huhnern. *Zentralb. f. Bakt. pt. I (Orig.)* 46, 595-609.

Fawcett, D. W. (1956). Electron microscope observations on intra-cellular virus-like particles associated with cells of the Lucké renal adenocarcinoma. *J. Biophys. Biochem. Cytol.* 2, 725-742.

Gross, L. (1951). Spontaneous leukaemia developing in C3H mice following inoculation in infancy with AL-leukaemic extracts or AK embryos. *Proc. Soc. exp. Biol Med.* 78, 27-32.

Heberling, R. L. and Kalter, S. A. (1978). Endogenous RNA viruses. *In* "Recent Advances in Primatology." (Chivers, D. J. and Ford, E. H. R., eds). pp. 87-97. London and N.Y.: Academic Press.

Hunt, R. D. (1978). Herpesvirus oncogenesis in New World monkeys: History of herpesvirus oncogenesis and overview of *Herpesvirus saimiri*. *In* "Recent Advances in Primatology." (Chivers, D. and Ford, E. H. R., eds). London and N.Y.: Academic Press.

Jarrett, W. F. H., Martin, W. B., Crighton, G. W., Dalton, R. G. and Stewart, M. F. (1964). Leukaemia in the cat. Transmission experiments with leukaemia (lymphosarcoma). *Nature* 202, 566-567.

Lucké, B. (1934). A neoplastic disease of the kidney of the frog (*Rana pipiens*). *Am. J. Cancer* 20, 352-379.

Lucké, B. (1938). Carcinoma in the leopard frog: its probable causation by a virus. *J. exp. Med.* 68, 457-468.

Melendez, L. V., Daniel, M. D., Hunt, R. D. and Garcia, F. G. (1968). An apparently new herpesvirus from primate kidney cultures of the squirrel monkey (*Saimiri sciureus*). *Lab. Anim. Care* 18, 374-381.

Melendez, L. V., Hunt, R. D., Daniel, M. D., Garcia, F. G. and Fraser, C. E. O. (1969). Herpes saimiri II. Experimentally induced malignant lymphoma in primates. *Lab. Anim. Care* 19, 378-386.

Melendez, L. V., Hunt, R. D., King, N. W., Barahona, H. H., Daniel, M. D. and Garcia, F. G. (1972). *Herpesvirus ateles*. A new lymphoma virus of monkeys. *Nature New Biol.* 235, 182-184.

Rous, P. (1911). A sarcoma of the fowl transmissible by an agent separable from the tumour cells. *J. exp. Med.* 13, 397-411.

Stewart, S. E. (1955a). Neoplasms in mice inoculated with cell-free extracts or filtrates of leukaemic mouse tissues. I. Neoplasms of the parotid and adrenal glands. *J. nat. Cancer Inst.* 15, 1392-1415.

Stewart, S. E. (1955b). Neoplasms of mice inoculated with cell-free extracts or filtrates of leukaemic mouse tissues. II. Leukaemia in hybrid mice produced by cell-free filtrates. *J. nat. Cancer Inst.* 16, 41-50.

Stewart, K. L., Snell, K. C., Dunham, L. C. and Schlyen, S. M. (1959). Transplantable and transmissible tumours of animals. Tumours of the kidney. Renal adeno-carcinoma. Frog. *In* "Atlas of Tumour Pathology." Sect. 12, Fasc. 40, Am. Reg. Path. Armed Forces Inst. Path., Washington, D.C.

Temin, H. and Mizutani, S. (1970). RNA-dependent DNA polymerase in virions of Rous Sarcoma virus. *Nature* **226,** 1211-1213.

Vizoso, A. D. (1970). Tumour viruses. *Proc. R. Soc. Med.* **63,** 341-344.

World Health Organization (1973). Immunity to cancer. *Bull. Wld Hlth Org.* **49,** 89-91; **49,** 205-213.

Index

DATE DUE